15–Minute Yoga

Chrissie Gallagher–Mundy

First published in 2007 by
Collins, an imprint of
HarperCollins Publishers
1 London Bridge Street,
London, SE1 9GF

www.collins.co.uk

Collins Gem is a registered
trademark of HarperCollins
Publishers Limited.

10 9 8 7 6 5

Text and photography
© HarperCollins

The copyright of the images
belongs to the following picture
libraries:

A catalogue record for this book
is available from the British
Library

Created by: SP Creative Design
Editor: Heather Thomas
Designer: Rolando Ugolini
Photographer: Ann Pownall

ISBN 13 - 9780007245628

Printed and bound in China by
RR Donnelley APS

Yoga can cause bodily injury so you should consult your doctor prior to
attempting any of the exercises contained in the book. The author and
publisher do not accept liability for any injury suffered as a result of
negligence in performing the exercises contained in this book. Exercises
contained in this book are carried out at your own risk and may not be
suitable for every reader.

CONTENTS

INTRODUCTION

Yoga is a great exercise and can be done by everyone. The way the body is taught to move in yoga is gentle yet challenging, logical yet improving and can benefit anyone who attempts it in a consistent way.

Ideally, yoga should be practised every day, and whilst this may not be practical for everyone, those devotees who do practise regularly will gradually notice differences and improvements to their bodies on a daily basis.

A HOLISTIC ACTIVITY

Yoga is a particularly interesting concept because it can be many different things to many people. On one level, it can be an effective form of exercise and a mode of keeping fit, whereas on another level, it can be a spiritual journey or, indeed, on yet a further level a full religious practice.

Those people who teach yoga undergo rigorous training, usually with old respected masters in India, and they are encouraged to take on all the different aspects of yoga as a complete way of thinking and living out their lives.

THE EIGHT LIMBS OF RAJA YOGA

According to the Sage Patanjali, the philosopher and founding father of yoga, there are eight limbs of Raja Yoga that form a series of steps to purifying the body and mind on its journey towards enlightenment. These steps are as follows:

Yama

This series of five moral codes exhorts truthfulness, non-violence, no stealing, non-possessiveness and moderation in all things. In many ways, it is similar in content and purpose to the Ten Commandments in Christianity).

Niyama

This is a set of five qualities to be sought and gained: purity, contentment, authority, awareness of the divine presence and study of the sacred texts.

Asanas

These are the postures and movements of the bodily being that are designed to extend, strengthen and keep the body fully flexible and able.

Pranayama

This is the next step on the road upwards: the study and use of the breath to aid mind and body.

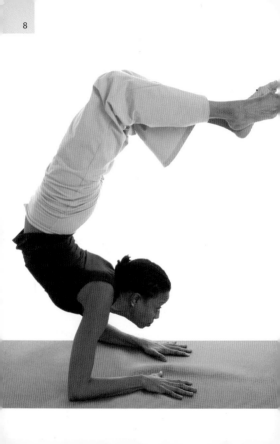

Pratyahara
This is the beginning of the study to gain control of the mind and become aware of its super-sensitivity to all around it.

Dharana
This is the first step toward concentration of the mind and beginning to tether it to certain areas at will.

Dhyana
This is a further stage of mind control with an effort to 'expand' the consciousness and to increase the sensitivity of the mind.

Samadhi
This is the final summit of mind, body and spirit control – the state of being at one with the creator or, in other words, transcendental bliss. This is personified in the act of contemplative sitting.

MOVEMENTS AND POSTURES

This book deals mainly with only one of the eight limbs of yoga: the asanas, or the movements and postures, on the third rung toward 'pure joy'. Some element of Pranayama (breathing) is also covered. For further and deeper study of yoga and all its elements please refer to page 189 for more information.

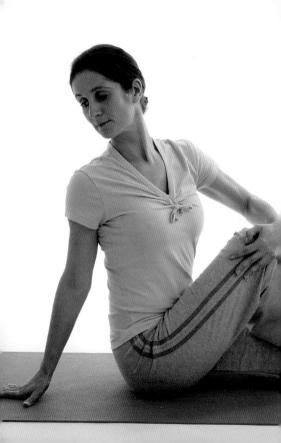

PART ONE

Getting started

The best way to get started with yoga is to begin! Start practising and learning the asanas (postures) and you will immediately begin to understand how yoga works on the body and the mind. Try to fit in a little yoga each day and you will soon notice the difference in your body, as it becomes more flexible and strong, and also your mind, as it becomes more focused.

HATHA YOGA

There are different ways to start the journey into yoga, but in Western society the route most often taken is the practice of Hatha Yoga. This term is used to describe the predominant study of the third and fourth limbs – the postures and breathing techniques.

AWARENESS OF BREATH

Once you begin to memorize and understand some of the postures, you will also learn to use the breath as directed, and utilize it as an aid to movement. This is where some of the magic of yoga will become apparent. In our modern society, we are unused to being aware of our breathing and using it to help us in our tasks. We mostly ignore the breath and what it can do for the body and often forget to breathe completely. How often have you held your breath when trying to do something challenging?

Power of breath

Hatha Yoga will teach you not only an awareness of breath but also a realization of its power to aid the body and quieten the mind. The asanas will give you an awareness of your body, how it works and how to strengthen and flex it, in a way you never knew existed.

PRACTICE IS IMPORTANT

The enlightenment of yoga begins with practice – there is no other way! All the Indian yogis agree on this and it really is true – by practising the asanas you will start to understand why all the hype about yoga is justified. As Sri K. Pattabhi Jois says: 'Do your practice and all is coming'.

GET IN THE MOOD

Start by finding an area in which to practise your yoga. Any space where you can lie full length and have some room on either side is fine. You can wear anything light and loose in which you can move easily. Bare arms are preferable, particularly for some of the more challenging positions.

HOW MUCH SPACE DO I NEED?

The ideal thing about yoga is that it does not take up a huge amount of space, unlike, say, aerobics or running, and you do not need basketfuls of equipment. You will need an area that is object free, well ventilated (as you will be sweating) and somewhere well away from noise and interruptions to allow your mind to concentrate on the task in

Mats, blocks and straps

As you progress in certain positions you may find it advantageous to have a foam block for support and a strap for facilitating stretching but that is all the equipment you will need besides your yoga mat which you can purchase online.

hand. A carpet can be used, but you may find that you slip on this, so a non-slip yoga mat is better.

LISTEN TO YOUR BREATHING

Unlike most other exercise, music or DVDs are not needed because you will be turning your focus inwards – onto your body and its breathing rhythms. You will be listening to your breathing and using this as your cue to move from position to position. As you progress, you will notice that your surroundings become less and less important as you become more focused on your movement and meditation.

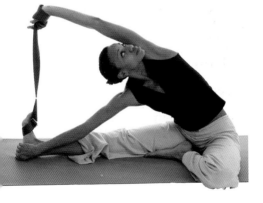

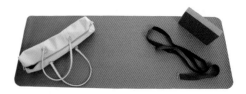

Yoga mats are now available in handy carry bags. Using blocks and straps will aid your yoga postures.

TIMING

A full yoga session can take in excess of one-and-a-half hours, but when you are starting out it is best to begin by practising short and often. Don't think that 10 minutes is not worth it because it is. One of the first sequences you will be learning is the Sun Salutations, and you can fit these into any time slot that you can make free in the course of a busy day.

Don't rush anything

Yoga is regulated by the breath, so if you perform it mindfully you won't be able to rush through any positions – it will take the time it takes. This is a useful first lesson for a stressed yoga novice!

FINDING A CLASS

Nowadays there are huge numbers of yoga classes available to the general public in gyms, health clubs and municipal centres. You can just turn up for most classes; the teacher should be able to accommodate you, whether you are a beginner or an advanced practitioner. If you do join a new class, do make sure that your teacher is aware of any injuries or physical problems you may have. This way, they can advise and enable you to work around any physical restrictions and even to help heal them.

It is important to choose the kind of class that suits you as there are many different ones. Below is a brief description of the more common classes available.

ASHTANGA YOGA

This form of yoga is very athletic and you jump from position to position. The second series of this type of yoga also involves gymnastics, including handstands, backward bends and some interesting extreme positions. A variant of this style of yoga is sometimes termed as 'Power Yoga'. You should not attempt this type of yoga unless you are very fit, active and flexible.

IYENGAR

Based on the teachings of Yogi B. K. S. Iyengar, this is one of the most popular forms of yoga. It favours holding the poses for much longer to develop the correct alignment and posture in each position.

KUNDALINI

This style uses the breath as the central part of the practice. Often the class will begin with chanting and there will be more deep exploration of the breath in relation to the movement.

BIKRAM

Bikram Yoga gets its name from its founding yogi Bikram Chouhouri, and is a set series of 26 postures that must be done in 40-degree heat. The idea of the

Individual tuition

Don't forget that you can also hire a teacher to work one-on-one with you. This may be beneficial at the beginning in helping to explain how to attempt some of the more complicated postures and how to use the breath to help you.

Yoga styles in this book

This book uses postures that come mainly from the Ashtanga and Iyengar styles of yoga, but you may also find them featured elsewhere.

heat is to focus the mind and loosen the body, along with sweating, which is thought to be detoxing. This form of yoga is sometime referred to as 'Hot Yoga'.

SIVANANDA

This form of yoga is more general, focusing on 12 poses along with periods of relaxation and breath work. This is a popular yoga form.

BEGINNING YOUR PRACTICE

To develop your practice to the point where it really makes a difference to your life and your body, try to do a little yoga every day. You need very little space, time or equipment, so there are no excuses.

The beauty of regular yoga practice is that you can begin to undergo a calming of the mind and an opening up of the body. This book will help you to experience the beginning of this breakthrough in movement and thought, and it will keep you challenged until you are ready to move on to a full series of postures.

HOW TO APPROACH YOUR PRACTICE

First of all, you must acquaint yourself with the different postures that you are going to perform at the beginning of each session. Most forms of yoga begin with the Sun Salutation series, and this is what you will focus on as your initial 'warm up'.

Start by learning, off by heart, the Sun Salutation A postures (see page 56). When you have mastered these, you can move on to the Sun Salutation B postures, approaching them in a similar way.

Guidelines

• Work through each move slowly, take your time and work on getting the movement right and feeling confident and balanced in each position – this may take several sessions.

• Don't worry about memorizing movements in the early stages – as you take time to work through each one, it will be absorbed into your body, so that you come to remember it.

• Then go back and work with the notes in this book to ensure you are performing the right breaths for the right movements. Each movement has an accompanying out or in breath (exhalation or inhalation). These are important because they help the body to achieve the linking movements and positions.

• Once you have learned the positions and their breath accompaniments you can start to move through the sequence as if it were a dance. Slowly progress, move by move, from one position to another in a seamless thread of movement.

• While you are doing this, concentrate your mind on perfecting each posture you move from and into. Use the notes in this book to focus on the aspects of the posture you should be working on.

• The beauty of the postures in yoga is that each one can be worked on indefinitely to achieve the perfect position, giving the mind something to think about with regard to the movement you are performing.

• You will discover, as you regularly practise Sun Salutation A, that your body will move in a rhythmic way as you work from posture to posture and your breath echos the rhythm. Your mind will be free from everyday thoughts as it focuses on each movement and how you should be doing it – when you should be breathing and which areas of muscle you should be contracting or extending.

• You will suddenly notice that you are moving, breathing and thinking in concert and almost subconsciously – that is the point at which you will begin to feel as though you are on another plane and almost meditating.

Build your practice

• Learn Sun Salutation A by heart.
• Learn Sun Salutation B by heart and add to A.
• Aim to learn two new yoga positions each day and add them to Sun Salutations A and B.

LEARNING OTHER POSTURES

After completing some warming up and 'meditating up' with the Sun Salutation series, you can move on to learning some other yoga postures. Work on these each day, and concentrate your efforts on mastering each new position and finding your way into it slowly.

Once you become familiar with each new move that you introduce, you can add it to the Sun Salutations, so that, once again, you are moving in a rhythmic and unconscious way and elongating your meditation moves.

CLOTHING AND EQUIPMENT

It is important to think about what you wear when doing yoga. Many of the positions involve placing a foot on the opposite leg, so some people prefer to keep their legs bare. There are also many twisting positions that necessitate wearing something soft and pliable – nothing with buckles, belts or pins.

Remember that when you start (it may be first thing in the morning), your body may be cold and therefore you may need to have several layers of soft, malleable clothing that you can shed as you warm up.

YOGA TROUSERS

Many specialist websites and shops sell yoga trousers. These are designed to be free flowing and wide legged to allow maximum movement. If you tend to get quite hot and sweaty – which you should do – bare flesh is always best. Wear shorts and a T-shirt made for exercise with breathable fabric underneath.

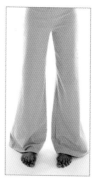

YOGA BLOCKS

The most helpful equipment apart from a yoga mat (see page 14) is a yoga block or brick. This is a solid foam block on which you place a hand or a foot to help you to balance if you cannot reach the full stretch in some positions. It allows you to balance a little further up the stretch, so you can work into the full positions in your own time.

YOGA STRAPS

Straps work in the same way as blocks to facilitate difficult positions but are used for those where you may be holding onto another body part. Therefore you can use the strap to wrap around a foot or wrist to help you work your way into the movement.

TEACHING AIDS

A wide range of DVDs is available to instruct you on all kinds of yoga. You can use these teaching aids to learn new moves and to discover different ways of getting into positions. Ultimately, however, you are still better off absorbing and learning the sequence of moves, so that you can fully get into your own rhythm and flow without having to rely on a television screen for instructions.

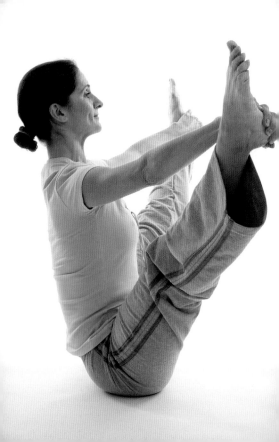

PART TWO

Body and mind

With Hatha Yoga providing such a strong
element of physical training, it is easy
to forget just how much of a body and
mind system yoga really is. There is a
strong connection between movement,
the breath and the mind to form the core
principles of yoga's path to enlightenment.
There is an assumption in yoga, which
initially was alien in the West, that the
mind and body are inextricably linked.

THE HISTORY OF YOGA

Yoga is a Sanskrit word meaning union, and it has always been about the process of spiritual and physical development. It has been traced back, in various forms, to its origins 5,000 years ago. Yoga poses have been discovered on stone seals dating from 3000 BC. However, some sources believe that it was introduced during the Stone Age along with Shamanism, and whilst latter-day yoga focuses on the development and enlightenment of the individual, it actually started out as a community-based activity to help people live happier lives.

Yoga has progressed through several periods: the Vedic, Pre-Classical, Classical and Post-Classical ones. It was during the Classical period that Pantajali systemized the steps toward Samadhi (see page 8), and in the Post-Classical period there is a proliferation of literature on yoga and its teachings.

WESTERN YOGA

Yoga was introduced into the West in the early nineteenth century and really began as a movement favouring healthy living and vegetarianism. However, it was not until the 1960s that the movement really became established. The Beatles helped to popularize it when they became interested in spirituality and wrote songs reflecting this. There was an influx of Indian yogis to England and America who spread their teachings together with more individual philosophies.

The Beatles' guru was Maharishi Mahesh, who was one of the first yogis to introduce transcendental meditation to the West. A doctor from Malaysia, Swami Sivananda, also became very well known, and he founded his own version of the yoga postures, known as Sivananda Yoga.

ASHTANGA YOGA

The Ashtanga yoga form was evolved by several yogis with its founding Yogi, Sri K. Pattabhi Jois being credited with the asanas as we now practise them. The original form may have come from the *Yoga Korunta*, a supposedly ancient manuscript written on palm leaves that has since disintegrated. This text passed through several yogis and was later passed down to Pattabhi Jois during the duration of his studies with Krishnamacharya, beginning in 1927.

The *Yoga Korunta* emphasized the importance of Vinyasa. This is breath-synchronized movement using the 'Ujjayi Pranayama'- a special breathing technique.

RECENT DECADES

The 1990s witnessed a huge interest and uptake of yoga in the West as aerobics lost its hold in the fitness world. Yoga seemed to offer a less competitive and more rounded and holistic approach to health. Many people are impressed by yoga's ability to make them strong – both mentally and physically – where more conventional exercise or medicine has failed.

Achieving enlightenment

The pro-active parts of yoga incorporate the asanas (postures), breath work, meditation and visualization, and are all concerned with harnessing the current of life force (prana). When this is practised, we can achieve Samadhi, or enlightenment. This is a state in which the body, mind and spirit are at one with the self and the outside universe – connected, blissful, aware yet serene.

THE BENEFITS OF YOGA

There are a great many benefits to be gained from following a yoga practice on a regular basis. As has already been described, yoga can be performed almost anywhere and with a minimum of specialist equipment, preparation or clothing.

Physiological benefits of yoga

Decreases:
- Body weight
- Pain
- Pulse rate
- Respiratory rate
- Blood pressure

Improves:
- Energy levels
- Endurance
- Muscular strength
- Lung efficiency
- Flexibility and movement ability
- Cardiovascular efficiency
- Respiratory efficiency
- Grip strength
- Immunity
- Galvanic skin response

May improve:
- Sleep
- Reaction time
- Dexterity
- Posture
- Balance
- Endocrine and gastrointestinal functions
- Autonomic nervous system

BOOKS ARE HELPFUL

Unlike most other forms of exercise during which there is no break or stop time, yoga is regulated by you and your breath, and therefore it is easier to follow yoga postures from a book. This way, they can be digested slowly and worked at gradually.

AGE AND COMPANY

No matter how old or how young you are, you can pursue the same goals of strength and suppleness and work in harmony together – or alone. When you

Psychological benefits

As well as the physical benefits derived from yoga, you may experience an improvement in:

- Mental performance
- Mood and vitality
- Self awareness
- Outlook

Other psychological benefits of practising yoga regularly include a decrease in:

- Panic attacks, which are often cured completely through
- the breath work
- Demotivation
- Anxiety

begin it may be beneficial to attend a class or hire a personal yoga teacher to oversee your moves, but you will soon feel more confident in working alone. The lists on page 31 and opposite show some of the benefits that you can expect to receive if you develop your yoga conscientiously.

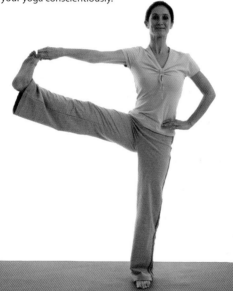

THE PHYSIOLOGY OF YOGA

Yoga is one of the most physiologically sound forms of movement in existence. Today, most osteopaths, chiropractors and physiotherapists recommend it as one of the more healing forms of exercise, and this is not to be taken lightly. They realize that yoga follows the basic laws and anatomy of the body to such an extent as to be beneficial, unlike some forms of exercise, which are essentially unnatural. An example of this is Classical ballet with its emphasis on unnatural alignment and extra turn-out in the hips and feet.

PRACTISING YOGA SAFELY

Some osteopaths become disillusioned when their surgeries fill up with over-zealous, impatient yoga devotees who force their knees, arms and feet into positions they are not ready for, thereby causing breaks and muscle pulls, so always practise safely.

Be safe and wise

If the yoga asanas are followed and developed wisely, a person can build strength, endurance and flexibility, safely and in a short period of time.

How to work the postures

It is important when you are starting out in yoga that you build up slowly. The emphasis from a good teacher will always be on the process – the means of developing the breath and movement – and not the achievement of the final position.

Twisting and binding

When it comes to twisting and binding (wrapping the limbs around the torso) there is a rule in yoga that one must attain the stretch before the binding is put in place. This approach means that each move is worked toward slowly and with control and awareness of breath.

Don't force a position

Never be tempted to try and force a position. Just hold the position for the number of breaths that is directed in the text, and during those breaths work to increase your ease in the position.

If you feel comfortable enough, you can stay in the position longer than the five breaths, but do not force anything or pull out of a position suddenly. The very act of having to breathe in time with each movement prevents a rushing of the moves, and gives you the time to move more deeply into each position. Work with your breath – not against it.

Don't rush your moves

In various positions you will note the direction to 'hold the position for five breaths'. This is to prevent you rushing or skimping over a move. The harder the move, the deeper and slower your five breaths will need to be to work and maintain the posture.

Another benefit of holding – and often struggling in – a posture, as you breathe, is that it builds heat. The hotter the inner body, the more flexibility you will achieve and the lower the risk of muscle pulls. As Beryl Bender Birch says: 'You have to be hot to stretch'.

Struggle to improve

Yoga is unique in its emphasis on holding, working and struggling within a position, and this brings so many benefits. For example, it won't take you long struggling with The Tree before you notice that your balance has significantly improved. Try this posture every day for a week and then try standing, casually on one leg to put your sock on.

You will be amazed at how much easier it is. It is this struggling that increases the body's strength. As you struggle and attempt to perform various postures, you will be realigning and balancing your body. You will develop more strength in one side as you discover an inequality on the other.

Stimulate and improve

There is another element that is unique to the yoga postures: in many of the positions you will be placing your heels or toes underneath another body part or twisting in such a way as to stimulate internal organs. These twisting and binding elements help to hinder the blood flow in one area and forward it to another.

For example, as you place a heel underneath your abdomen and lean forward, you will be stimulating your internal digestion. As you twist and bend your spine both forward and backward, you will stimulate it, flex it and keep it healthy. So think of yoga as an all-round health improvement.

Holistic balance

The heat and work you put into trying to develop a position will align your body, strengthen and stretch your muscles, and focus your mind.

BREATHING

Breathing forms one of the most central tenets of the yoga tradition and, as such, should be studied in its own right alongside the postures. Yoga breathing involves a whole science of breath control of which non-practitioners are not aware. According to the gurus from India, Western breathing is not as helpful as it should be to our health and well-being.

TYPES OF BREATHING

There are three types of breathing:
• Clavicular breathing (breathing shallowly, only into the chest area)
• Intercostal breathing (into the middle rib cage area)
• Abdominal breathing (deeper and more complete)

A full breath in yoga would consist of all three types of breathing, starting with the deep breath into the abdomen and then continuing up through the rib cage into the chest.

Yogis claim that many people have forgotten how to breathe properly with the result that they breathe only into the chest area, through their mouth without involving the diaphragm.

In yoga, you will learn how to develop your breathing to a greater level, so that you will be exercising and working your diaphragm and your nostrils, thereby taking in more oxygen more efficiently.

LEARNING TO BREATHE PROPERLY

Breathing correctly means using your entire torso to inhale and exhale the air. It involves breathing though the nose and making a full inhalation and exhalation with the whole of the lungs. When you do this, the abdomen aids the exhalation and moves the diaphragm up, massaging the heart. As it moves down, it massages the abdominal organs.

EXERCISE FOR BASIC BREATHING

Sit cross-legged in the Half Lotus (see page 87) on the floor. This strengthens and straightens the back, allowing better air flow. Sitting hunched up over a computer or book rounds the back, curves the chest (which houses the important lungs) and cramps the abdominal section. There are three parts to a full breath: the inhalation, a hold and an exhalation.

1 Breathe in through your nose slowly. Allow the breath to travel down until you feel it swelling your abdominal section. Once this happens, keep inhaling until your breath fills the rib cage and finally lifts the chest. Hold this position for a moment.

2 Slowly exhale the air from your lungs, mindfully and using the abdominal muscle to continue expelling the air until you feel it has all gone. Your abdominal muscles will be contracted and pulled in, and you will notice that your exhalation takes longer than normal.

Awareness of breath

This is what a full breath feels like. Most of the time our breath is unconscious and we don't spend time

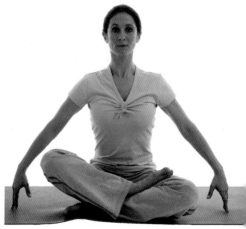

thinking of the mechanics. However, when we are doing yoga we can take time to become aware of our greater powers of oxygenating, so that when we need it our breath can aid us greatly.

Controlling your mind

When you regulate and focus on your breathing you become aware of another element. You are beginning to control your mind. It cannot wander if you count and control your breath as it takes your full consciousness to achieve this. This is the start of your meditative skills.

OTHER BREATHING EXERCISES

In addition to the basic breathing already described, you can practise the following methods.

'Skull shining' method

This method of breathing (Kapalahabhati) helps to increase the amount of oxygen in the body, clearing the mind and aiding concentration.

1 Start by sitting in the Half Lotus (see page 87) with your wrist resting on your knees and the forefinger and thumb lightly touching.
2 Take two normal breaths.
3 Inhale, expanding your abdomen.
4 Exhale, pulling in your abdomen.

CLEANSING THE RESPIRATORY SYSTEM
The exhalation should be short and audible; the inhalation can be longer and silent. Repeat 20 times; keep a steady rhythm, but make the exhalation forceful. After 20 repetitions, inhale and exhale, then inhale and hold the breath for as long as you can before slowly exhaling. Begin by practising three rounds of 20 pumpings and then build up to 60. This technique is thought to rid stale air from the lungs, allowing fresh oxygen-rich air in and cleansing the respiratory system.

Blocking off one nostril

This method (Anuloma Viloma) involves the blocking off of one nostril and then the other. The left nostril is believed to be the path of the nadi called Ida, while the right nostril is the path of Pingala.

Yogis believe that if you are healthy you breathe from the left nostril predominantly for a period and then through the right one. They think that in many people this rhythm has become disturbed, and this exercise serves to restore the balance.

1 Sit in the Lotus (see page 88) or Half Lotus position (see page 87) with a straight back.
2 Place your right hand in the position that is shown opposite. The Vishna mudra is a hand position with

your index and middle fingers tucked into your palm. When you lift your hand, you place the fingers and thumb either side of the nose.

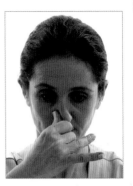

3 Now place the thumb to close off the right nostril, with the first and second finger tucked into the palm.

4 Breathe in through the left nostril for a count of 4.

5 Hold the breath for 16 counts (press the last fingers and thumb to close off both nostrils).

6 Open the right nostril and breathe out through it for a count of 8, while closing off the left nostril with the last two fingers

7 Breathe in through the right nostril for a count of 4.

8 Hold the breath for 16 counts (closing both nostrils).

9 Breathe out through the left nostril (closing off the right with the thumb) to a count of 8.

Note: This exercise will take some practice, but once you have mastered the sequence it is thought to bring prana (life force) up through the body. Start by practising three rounds and build up to 20.

BANDHAS

These are a very important part of the physical practice of yoga and help to make the movements easier and lighter. They are thought to aid the prana's progress up through the body and to stimulate energy and lift. The bandhas are a kind of 'lock' or contraction that you use to provide a solid base for muscle work and to prevent prana from seeping away.

MOOLA BANDHA

This bandha is called 'root lock' and provides a strong pelvis for movement of the body and its energy. It is all about contracting the pelvic floor muscles and the lower abdominals. Pull up the muscles that you might use when going to the bathroom and pull in your lower stomach. This produces heat (which enables muscle movement) and concentrates the mind.

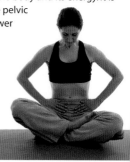

UDDIYANA BANDHA

A dynamic bandha, this is known as 'upward flying'. It can be practised in the Downward Dog position (see page 61) where you remain for five breaths. Be aware of the diaphragm relaxing and the drawing in of the abdominal muscles at the end of an exhalation.

You can practise this bandha standing as you draw the navel inward and upward, lifting the whole torso – toning it and making it ready for action. It creates heat and readiness for movement and energy, and also strengthens and tones the internal organs of the pelvic region.

Energy flow

Despite their 'locking' effect, the bandhas release energy through the body and direct it upward, helping concentration, energy flow and tranquillity.

MEDITATION

Meditation is really about stilling the mind. We all know the feeling when our mind races around different ideas, thoughts, concerns and worries and gives us little peace. We also recognize when we are focused on an absorbing task and suddenly realize our mind has slowed down and we are feeling more at ease. Meditation (or the first stage – concentration) is the journey toward a more focused mind that can concentrate on the task in hand and, ultimately, on our inner self – so we can feel the wisdom and tranquillity within. We can also experience the wider universe without being distracted by our own ego.

When we begin to harness the mind a little, we can stop the constant chattering in our head and the brain skipping from one subject to another – that is when we can begin to experience real peace.

CONCENTRATION

This is the first level of meditation where we train the mind to focus on a specific object and not to be distracted by anything else. When you begin this initial stage, you may find it hard: it is sometimes difficult to stop your mind wandering from one concern to another, and you may have to keep pulling it back to the object on which you are trying to focus. Concentration will take practice and is an active use of your brain.

The Solar System

Try this exercise to begin concentrating the mind.

1 Sit quietly and try to clear your mind. Think of nothing; be warned – this is extremely difficult. The way to do this is to try and imagine that your mind is like a solar system –dark black and with nothing in it.
2 As, inevitably, you start to get different thoughts encroaching across this blank canvas, allow them to come but do not follow them.
3 Watch your thoughts come and go, as if they are stars whizzing across your solar system, but do not follow a thought and get caught up in its detail.
4 Slowly, you will notice that you can become a spectator of your own thoughts – watching them coming and going but not following them or being affected by them.

Serenity

You will feel much calmer and more serene after completing a meditation session like this.

Concentration during the asanas

You can also use this method when doing your asanas – try to concentrate purely on the movement you should be doing, the breathing you should be using and the gaze you should direct. Think also about your bandhas – by the time you have thought of all these things as you move, you won't have time for your mind to wander.

FULLER MEDITATION

When you have mastered the first level – the concentration stage – you can progress to the second level, which is a fuller meditation. The mind will become still and you do not have to work so consciously to keep it in check.

Mantras

Meditators often work with mantras, images or objects to help give their mind a focus.

Types of meditation

There are conventionally two types of meditation: Saguna and Nirguna.

• Saguna is where you imagine yourself sitting at the centre of a sphere (this represents the absolute) and use the mantras, images or objects to still the mind.

• In Nirguna meditation, you move beyond the focus of the object to a greater awareness of the universe.

The basic meditation routine

Start your meditation by sitting somewhere cool, but not cold, where you will not be disturbed. Choose a time when your mind will not be filled with thoughts and worries about work or other issues and when you have time to devote to your meditative task.

1 Sit in a restful posture and keep your back straight.

2 Focus on your breathing, becoming aware of it and working to slow it down and regulate it, if necessary.

3 Start to elongate your breaths, so you are taking

Pure bliss

Meditation is thought to be in place when your mind will stay with the focus of its own accord and you are freed of normal everyday thoughts. With long practice, the state of Samadhi is said to be achieved – pure bliss!

longer inhalations and even longer exhalations.
4 Allow your mind to wander as you establish the breathing pattern, and then slowly try to focus on the object or mantra of your choice.
5 Try to hold the object as the centre of your thoughts. Return the mind each time it tries to wander, and keep the breath steady and rhythmical.

MEDITATION POSITIONS

You can choose to sit in any position for meditation but the Lotus, Half Lotus or Easy Poses work best. In these positions, you are balanced with the back and torso straight to aid digestion and deep breathing. These positions and how to adopt them are described in detail later on in the book (see page 86). Few beginners could achieve the Full Lotus position but they may be flexible

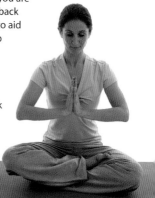

enough to manage the Half Lotus. However, if this requires more flexibility than you currently have, you can try the Easy Pose (see page 166).

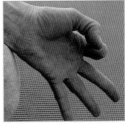

Chin Mudra

You can rest your wrists on your knees and group your hands into 'Chin Mudra', which is thought to help focus the mind, too. To do this, stretch your hands out and press your thumb and first finger together, the nail under the thumb (as shown in the photograph above).

BENEFITS OF MEDITATION

It will take time and practice but true meditation will benefit you greatly. As you learn to train the mind, you can free yourself of many everyday irritants and worries, refreshing your mind like you would refresh your body after a cool swim. You will come to realize that your mood emanates from within and that you can remain calm even with daily changes in circumstance. You will learn that we possess the power to be happy outside of material possessions and the material world.

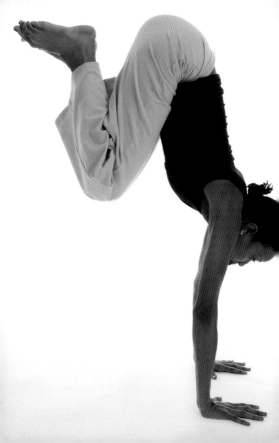

PART THREE

The Sun Salutations

The Sun Salutations are a great way to start your yoga programme and develop good habits for your practice. They are comprised of two sequences, which are similar in nature and which build into a steady rhythmical set of movements that will get you into the 'flow'.

WARMING UP

Think of the Sun Salutations as your warm-up period for yoga practice. While you bend and arch, you will build up the heat in your body that will enable you to work on more advanced postures later in the session.

However, the Sun Salutations are not just a warm-up; they are also a set of excellent exercises in their own right. They serve to mobilize the whole body, bending the spine both backwards and forwards and readying the arms for weight and the legs for stretching.

They allow you time to focus the breathing, so that you are using the breath with each movement and exhaling and inhaling strongly and lengthily to further prolong the movement.

TAKE YOUR TIME

When you begin your first flow through the postures of the Sun Salutations, you may well feel a little stiff (particularly if you are doing your practice in the morning) and the movements may be quite jerky. However, don't worry about this – just take your time and move around as well as you can. Remember that yoga practice builds – it builds heat, rhythm and suppleness in the body. Therefore don't become discouraged but simply keep moving.

BUILDING A ROUTINE

You will need to repeat the Sun Salutations A and B as many times as you can to begin with. Try starting with five A routines followed by three B routines.

As you get stronger, you should try to increase to doing 10 Sun Salutation A's and five Sun Salutation B's. This will not only build strength and suppleness but will also allow you to thoroughly absorb the rhythm of the movement.

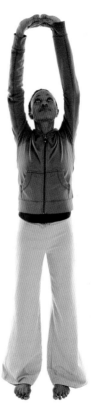

Reaching and extending the limbs invigorates and warms the body

SUN SALUTATION A

Many of the standing postures in yoga and the Sun Salutation sequences all start with the Mountain pose, or the Tadasana pose as it is sometimes called.

MOUNTAIN POSE

1 Stand with your feet together with your arms by your sides.
2 Look down and check that your heels, ankles and big toes are all touching.
3 Now lift up through your body as though there is a string pulling the top of your head – elongating your whole spine upward.
4 Check your shoulders – they should be neither forward nor pushed falsely back, but you should feel them dropping down, down behind you.
5 Pull in and up on the stomach area, so your rib

Good posture

This pose alone will help to improve your posture and body alignment. It helps teach you to stand in a balanced and supported way that will breed good postural habits.

cage feels lifted, allowing space underneath for the digestion.

6 Pull up your knee caps to tighten the quadriceps muscles on the thighs.

7 Now think about your coccyx (the bone at the base of the spine). It should be pointed down towards the floor, not tilting toward the back of the room. This will ensure that your hips and your pelvis are in the right place.

8 Finally, feel your feet pressing into the ground on the heels and toes, and think about contracting the arches of each foot to keep them toned.

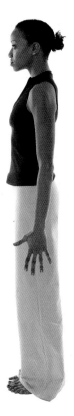

STEP 1

1 Inhale on this move. Lift both arms outwards and bring them together, touching your palms together above your head.
2 Reach upwards as strongly as you can, really trying to lift up through your torso. Don't lift your shoulders and arch backwards too far.

STEP 2

1 Exhale on this move. Keep reaching with your arms and allow them to lean you forwards from the hips as you take your hands down towards the floor.
2 Keep your knees pulled up and abdominals (the bandha lock, see page 44) contracted as you bend forwards.
3 Place your hands on the floor on either side of your feet. If you can't do this with your legs straight, bend your knees – as much as it takes – until you can place your hands down.

STEP 3

1 Inhale on this move. Lift your head to look up and out, pulling your shoulder blades back to avoid the shoulders rounding.
2 Keep your hands on the floor and, if you can, your legs straight. If your legs need to stay bent, that's fine – you can still extend your back. Aim to lengthen your spine from the base to the neck.

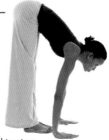

STEP 4

1 Exhale on this move. Walk your feet back until your body is in a straight plank with your hands and toes on the floor – the classic push-up position.
Taking it further: As you become more flexible, try jumping your feet back into this pose.
2 Bend your arms and lower your body until it is just off the floor. If you don't have the strength, lower your knees to the ground to help. This is the 'Four Limbed Stick Posture'.

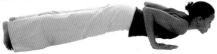

STEP 5

1 Inhale on this move. Roll over your toes to flatten the top of the feet on the floor.
2 Press your hips forwards and lift your chest to arch up and back.
Taking it further: Raise your thighs and hips off the floor and keep your arms straight. If this is difficult, keep your knees on the floor and your arms a little bent.

STEP 6

1 Exhale to get into this move, then remain in this posture for 5 breaths.
2 Lift your hips strongly upwards and roll back over your toes to press your heels towards the floor. Your weight will be on your hands and feet. This is known as 'Downward Dog'.

3 While doing 5 breaths, try to press your armpits towards the floor, extending the shoulders; don't forget to squeeze your shoulder blades together.
4 Tilt your hips towards the ceiling as if trying to press your hip bones against your thighs.

STEP 7

1 Inhale into this position. Step one foot in towards your hands and bring the other foot underneath you.
Taking it further: Jump both feet from Downward Dog right between your hands.
2 Now lift your back again and straighten your legs as much as you can. Be sure to keep your fingertips on the floor.
Note: This is the same position as Step 3.

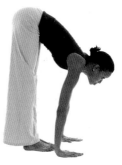

STEP 8

1 Exhale in this position. Press your head in towards your knees. Do not forget to pull up on your knees at all times when your legs are straight.
2 If you need to bend your knees, that's fine – you can still pull your head in.
3 In this position, you are looking at your navel.

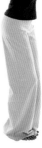

STEP 9

1 Inhale in this position. Lift your body and arms up to the ceiling to finish in the same position as Step 1.
2 Use this position to end the Sun Salutation A sequence and also to prepare yourself for the next round.

SUN SALUTATION B

Sun Salutation B is a very similar sequence to Sun Salutation A, but with added positions. Once you are accustomed to working through Sun Salutation A, doing B will feel natural, although it is hard work.

WORKING YOUR WHOLE BODY

The Sun Salutations work practically all of your body, bending it forwards and backwards and warming up the back and front superior muscles. When you progress to other positions, you will also be working the side muscles and the inner inferior muscles.

You should progress gradually and concentrate on mastering (and learning by heart) the Sun Salutation B sequence. Start off as normal with the reach upwards and forwards, but as you come out of the Downward Dog position, turn your foot and move into the Warrior position – a pose in its own right, which you will learn later on (see page 96). Move from this into the final Downward Dog posture and then onto the finishing postures. You should try to learn this sequence, as you have learned Sun Salutation A, and don't forget to keep count as you work through 5–10 repetitions.

STEP 1

1 Stand in the Mountain pose to start (see page 56). Exhale in this position. Bend your knees and lift your arms up above your head.
2 Keep your shoulders pressed down and feel the stretch in the shoulder area as you look upwards.
3 Keep your knees pulled together and try to think of your bandhas.

STEP 2

1 Inhale as you go into this position. Straighten up from your bend and then lean forwards slowly to take your hands down to the floor – you can bend your knees if you need to, as you did with Sun Salutation A.
2 Press your head down towards your knees.

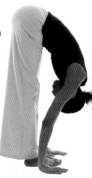

STEP 3

1 Inhale on this move. Lift your head to look up and out, pulling your shoulder blades back to avoid the shoulders rounding.
2 Keep your hands on the floor and your legs straight. If they need to stay bent, that's fine – you can still extend them back. Lengthen your spine from the base to your neck.

STEP 4

1 Exhale on this move. Walk your feet back until your body is in a straight plank with your hands and toes on the floor.
2 Bend your arms and lower your body until it is just off the floor. If you don't have the strength to do this, lower your knees to the ground to help. This position is called the 'Four Limbed Stick Posture'.

STEP 5

1 Inhale on this move. Roll over your toes to flatten the top of your feet on the floor.
2 Press your hips forward and lift your chest to arch up and back. If you find this difficult, keep your knees on the floor and your arms a little bent.
Taking it further: Try to lift your thighs and hips off the floor; keep your arms straight.

STEP 6

Exhale to get into this move – the Downward Dog position (see page 60). Unlike Sun Salutation A, you will not be holding this position yet.

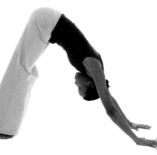

STEP 7

1 Inhale as you negotiate this position. Turn your left heel, so it is at right angles to the right, with the heel pointing towards the toes.
2 Lift your foot and place it between your hands. When you first attempt this, it may seem impossible, but keep on trying every day and it will eventually happen. For now, just bring your foot as near as you can.
3 Lift your arms over your head and look upwards.

STEP 8

1 Exhale in this position. Move your arms back to the floor and your leg back, so you can lower into a push-up position.
2 Now lower yourself down even further.

STEP 9

1 Inhale on this move. Roll over your toes to flatten the top of your feet on the floor.
2 Press your hips forward and lift your chest to arch it up and back.
Taking it further: Lift your thighs and hips off the floor, with arms straight. If this is difficult, keep your knees on the floor and your arms a little bent.

STEP 10

1 This position is back into Downward Dog. You need to lift your hips strongly upwards and roll back over your toes to press the heels towards the floor.
2 Your weight is on your hands and your feet.

STEP 11

1 Inhale as you negotiate this position. Turn the right heel, so it is at right angles to the left, with the heel pointing towards the toes.
2 Lift your foot and place it between your hands. If you can't manage this, just bring the foot as near as you can.
3 Lift your arms over your head and look and stretch upwards.

STEP 12

1 Exhale in this position. Move your arms back to the floor and your leg back, so that you can lower yourself into a push-up position.
2 Now lower yourself down further.

STEP 13

1 Inhale on this move – the Face Up Dog.
Roll over your toes to flatten the top of
your feet on the floor.
2 Press your hips forwards and lift your
chest to arch up and back.
Taking it further: Lift your thighs and
hips off the floor, with arms straight. If
difficult, keep your knees on the floor
and your arms a little bent.

STEP 14

1 This is back into
Downward Dog. Lift
your hips strongly
upwards and roll
back over your
toes to press your
heels towards
the floor.
2 Exhale to get
into this move. Remain in the posture for 5 breaths.

STEP 15

1 Inhale into
this position.
Step one foot in
towards your hands
and bring the other
foot underneath you.
Taking it further: Jump both
feet from Downward Dog right
between your hands.
2 Lift your back again and straighten
your legs as much as you can with your
fingertips on the floor. This is the same
position as in Step 3.

STEP 16

1 Exhale in this position. Press
your head in towards your
knees. Don't forget to pull
up on your knees at all times
when your legs are straight.
2 If you need to bend your
knees, that's fine – you can still
pull your head in. In this position,
you are looking at
your navel.

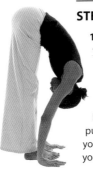

STEP 17

1 Inhale in this position. Lift your torso up and lift your arms up to the ceiling.

2 This is the same position as Step 1, so bend your knees and stretch fully upward with arms overhead before finally returning to the Mountain posture (see opposite and page 56).

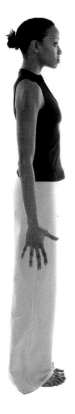

Eating and drinking

After your yoga practice, drink some cool water and then wait for a while before you eat anything. This is rather like the 'cool down' period that is suggested in many other forms of exercise and really just allows the body some healing time after the stress of the main work-out.

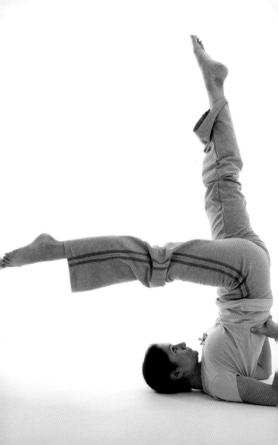

PART FOUR

Closing sequences

In most yoga disciplines there is a set way to approach the practice. The postures are aligned in a specific order to develop the stretch and strength of the body, and it is best to keep to this order, if you possibly can. In Ashtanga Yoga, there is a 'closing sequence' which is believed to bring the body back to its normal state after the main practice and allow the system to return to neutral.

COOLING DOWN

At the end of any exercise, it is important to have
a cooling down period, and yoga provides its own
version. The position most often used is the Corpse,
or relaxation, pose. Use this as the final posture of
your work-out to allow your body to absorb some
of the stretching changes you have made. When
you perform the closing sequence postures, you
will notice the calmness creeping into your system,
making you ready for anything in your day.

SAFETY FIRST

With many of the postures in this book, there are
times when the positions may be challenging. Yoga
requires you to listen to your body and assess what
it can take. No one else can feel what you are feeling,
and only you can judge whether you are pushing
yourself too far. Just breathe into the position and
then maintain it if you can.

Yoga is not competitive – it is a meditative exercise –
so you should not feel that you have to keep pushing
further and further. Take your time with each posture
and don't worry if you don't attain it on day one.
If you keep practising, you will achieve it one day.

CORPSE

1 Lie on the floor and allow your feet to fall outwards.
2 Rest your arms on the floor away from your body with the palms of the hands facing upwards.
3 Breathe normally and look straight up.
4 Now allow your body to really 'fall into' and rest on the floor – feel the weight of your pelvis sinking, the weight of your buttocks, the weight of your shoulder blades, and so on.
5 Particularly try to notice the weight of your head sinking into the floor, so that your neck really relaxes.
6 Stay in this position until all the aches from your practice have receded, then slowly bring yourself up to a sitting position and then gradually roll up into a standing position.

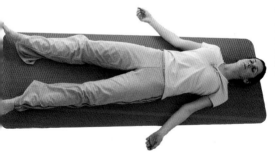

SHOULDER STAND

The Shoulder Stand is a great way of ending a yoga work-out session. It is believed to stimulate the thyroid gland because of its weight emphasis on the neck. It also brings blood to the head and neck, which is not something we achieve very often.

1 Lie on the floor with your legs and arms straight.
2 Bend your knees and lift your legs and hips off the floor and up into the straight position.
3 Keeping your head facing forwards, balance on your shoulders, using your hands for support.
4 Remain in this position for up to 20 breaths.

Warning

Avoid using this position if you have bad neck problems until you can get expert supervision from a qualified teacher.

Getting into the Shoulder Stand

The Shoulder Stand can be a challenging position to get into if you are not accustomed to turning upside down – but don't panic! As you keep on practising these positions, they will become easier to negotiate.

For the lift into the Shoulder Stand you need to have built up your lower abdomen strength – do this as you practise the bandhas and other postures.

STAGE 1: REVERSE CURLS

This is actually a stomach toning exercise but will help you in your preparation for the Shoulder Stand.

1 Lie on your back and bend your knees, pressing your hands to the floor.
2 Contract the lower abdomen, activate your bandhas and try to lift your hips off the floor. Do not swing your knees; focus on contracting the lower abdomen.
3 Perform 15–20 repetitions to build up strength in this area.

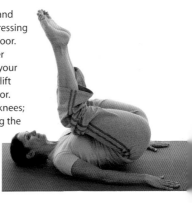

STAGE 2

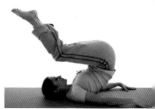

1 Lie on your back with arms by your sides, palms facing the floor and legs stretched out on the floor.

2 Activate your bandhas and bend your legs, bringing your knees in towards your chest and contracting your lower abdominals to boost your hips off the ground and direct your feet towards your head.

3 Place your hands behind your hips to support yourself and hold the position just for a moment. Then release with control.

STAGE 3

Now that you are able to boost your hips off the floor and lift your legs over your head, try to straighten your body more. You need to get the weight of your body further onto your shoulders and point your toes with a vengeance towards the ceiling. Try to hold this pose for several breaths.

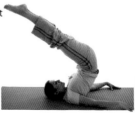

PLOUGH

Once you have attempted the Shoulder Stand, you can try this position. It will stretch your neck, backs of shoulders, upper back and backs of legs. Try to remain in the position for 5 breaths. Build up gradually by holding the position for 2 breaths, and the next time you attempt it hold it a little longer and so on until you can remain comfortably for 5 full breaths.

1 Begin from the Shoulder Stand. From the full position, lower your legs slowly behind your head.
2 Touch your toes to the floor behind you if you can.
3 Reach your arms out behind you and clasp your hands together. Remain for 5 breaths.

Note: Avoid this position if you have bad neck problems until you can get supervision from a qualified yoga teacher.

PRESS THE EAR POSTURE

This posture follows on from the last posture, so note the logic of doing the postures in the correct order.

1 From the previous posture, simply bend your knees, so that, ideally, they slide by the side of each ear.
2 Hold this position for 5 breaths.
3 If your knees won't touch your ears, just stay in the position as best you can and breathe. Avoid this position if you have bad neck problems until you can get advice from a qualified teacher.

It's worth the struggle

As with all these positions you may find you have to struggle a little. This is what yoga is all about! The struggle to maintain and attain a position will strengthen and stretch you each day.

HEADSTAND

This is another great posture that brings blood to the head and neck and will really work all your postural muscles. As you learn to maintain your balance in the stand, you will be working small and large muscles throughout your torso. You will notice the benefits of this as you continue to practise: you will feel more balanced and stronger throughout your normal day. The weight placement of the Headstand should be on the arms as much as the head, so you will be toning and strengthening the shoulders and arms, too.

Safety

Throwing your legs up in the air can seem a scary prospect if you haven't done it since you were a child. Don't worry – you are going to go into this gradually. You may find it easier to place a mattress on the floor when you first try this to ease your fear of falling.

FALLING

If you do over-balance, simply unlock your fingers and tuck your head under into a roll as you fall over. If it seems easier, you can fall and arch with one foot coming onto the floor, then the other. These actions will be instinctive if and when it happens. The other way is to place your balance next to a wall; that way, if you over-balance you will just touch the wall.

Headstand preparation

1 Start by placing your hands and head in a triangle shape on the floor. When you begin, use a soft towel, folded under your head, to take the weight. Place the top of your head, towards the forehead, on the floor.

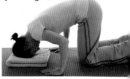

2 Using your feet, walk your bottom into the air and bring your hips up and over your shoulders. Hold this position to absorb how the weight feels on your head.

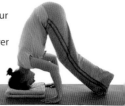

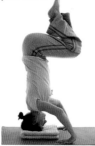

3 Now, if you can, push your hips a little further forward and try and just kick your feet off the ground into a balance. Do keep practising this until you feel comfortable. If you are worried about falling over, then practise the stand against a wall.

Headstand practice

1 In yoga, the arms are placed in different positions from the exercise opposite. Start on your knees and lean forwards to place your elbows, with the hands folded across, on the floor. Inhale.

2 Release your hands and clasp them in front of you to form a triangle.

3 Place your head in the triangle with the crown touching the floor.

4 Walk your feet in to lift your hips, and keep walking in your toes until you can lift them off the floor. Exhale.

Taking it further: Roll over your toes and then lift your feet.

5 If you can, lift your legs just off the ground and hold for 5 breaths, then return your feet to the floor. If you tip your hips enough, you should feel your feet lift automatically; soon you will be able to lever your legs even higher.

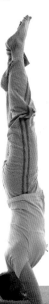

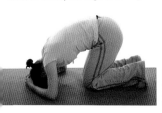

LOTUS POSITIONS

To end your practice you will need to use one of the Lotus positions. This is the classic yoga pose that is associated with Yogis and their teachers, but don't be fooled – you still need a good degree of flexibility to get into this position. You will need to build up to it gradually, like all the other postures.

SAFETY

Do not be tempted to force your legs into the Lotus postures as you could damage your feet or ankles. The flexibility will come from your hips as your legs loosen up, allowing you to position your foot in the right place. Opposite you can see that the model's right knee is off the floor. As her flexibility improves, however, the knee will rest on the floor.

HALF LOTUS

1 Sit with one leg bent underneath you.
2 Begin by loosening the hips: take hold of one of your legs and cradle it in your arms.
3 Hold the ankle and the foot with both hands and gently move the leg round in a circle in order to mobilize the hip.

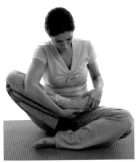

4 Now press your knee away from you as you attempt to position the back of your foot on your thigh.
5 Try to place the heel of the foot in towards the stomach area just above the opposite hip.
6 Aim to sit upright and your knee should fall down towards the floor – breathe for 5 breaths.

FULL LOTUS

As your hips loosen, you can attempt the Full Lotus, but remember not to force it – mobilize it. This may take you some time to achieve.

1 Bend your right leg and rest the foot on your thigh.
2 Now take your left leg and cross it over – you may need to inch the foot over the other shin slowly – and place your left foot on your right leg.
3 When you have achieved this properly, you will feel that the position is stable.
4 Release the left leg to release yourself from the position. When you are ready, you can begin building up to 20 breaths in this position.

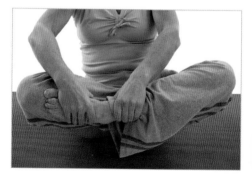

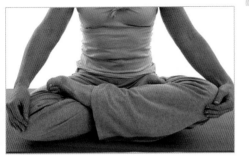

Build up gradually

Always attempt the Full Lotus when you are really warm, and your ankles, knee joints and hips have been loosened up. You may only be able to hold the Lotus for a short time when you are starting your yoga practice, but as you progress you can build up to sitting in the position for 100 breaths – or while you are watching television.

Flexibility is essential

The Full Lotus may feel quite uncomfortable at first, as this position requires not just flexibility in your hips but also in your ankles. Don't forget to pull up on your bandhas and take deep breaths.

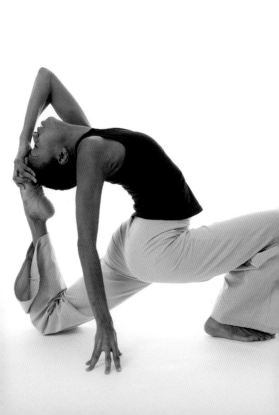

PART FIVE

15-minute wake-up routine

Every day, break your yoga practice up into several timed sections. Fifteen minutes is an ideal time slot as it fits into most days yet is long enough to make progress. When you wake up in the morning, your body may not be at its most flexible and trying some of the postures will feel very challenging – don't be put off! This is all part of the yoga mission: struggling against a difficulty, building heat and gaining strength and flexibility.

STARTING YOUR PRACTICE

What the morning practice will do for you is wake you up in a really fundamental way – inside and out – and ready you for any action needed in your day. You will notice after your morning practice that you will feel more confident, more prepared and more optimistic about the day ahead of you.

It is not always easy to do your yoga practice first thing in the morning. You may be surprised to learn that the posture you struggle with on waking up will seem a lot easier later on in the day. However, that does not mean you should avoid the mornings; just do your 15-minute practice early knowing that you are up against your body's natural stiffening after a night's sleep.

SUN SALUTATIONS

Always start with the Sun Salutations. In the morning even these may test you, but repeat enough of both A (see page 56) and B (see page 63) until you feel warm and awake. These are important to ready your body for further postures as well as synchronizing your breathing. When you are warmed up and wide awake, you can embark on the following positions.

DOWNWARD DOG DETAIL

You have already performed Downward Dog as part of your Sun Salutation sequence (see page 60) but now you are going to take it a little further.

1 Come onto your hands and knees and press from here into the Downward Dog. Stay like this for up to 10 breaths and really work the position.

2 Press your arm pits towards the floor to flex the shoulder joints. Keep inhaling and exhaling long breaths.

3 As you work your shoulders, pull the shoulder blades back together and feel the outside of the shoulders rounding back. Keep your neck lengthened but look towards your navel.

4 Try to press your heels to the floor (this may not happen on the first breath). Check the outside of the heels and legs are being pressed down.

5 To work the lower body further, try to press your lower stomach towards the top of your thighs. This way you are extending the stretch in your lower back and the backs of the legs.

BENEFITS OF DOWNWARD DOG

There are a great many benefits to all the postures in yoga, especially in those that are done in a specific order that first stretches one part, then another. Downward Dog is a great pose for a wake-up session.

• It helps loosen the whole of the back of the body and aids mobility in the shoulders, hips and backs of legs.
• It helps back and shoulder problems. If you feel any extreme pain, then rest and retry. Strong pains in the backs of the legs are common in people with tight hamstrings; as you practise this (and other positions)

Check

• Have you contracted your pelvic floor and transverse abdominals to form the bandha lock?
• Are you still taking deep long breaths?
• Are you still focusing on your navel?

By the time you have worked your way through these check points you should have performed at least 10 breaths and yet your mind will not have wandered at all. This is all part of the yoga experience: as you concentrate on what you are doing physically, your mind is reined in mentally.

regularly they will start to recede. Don't push yourself further than what feels right as you breathe.

• This posture lengthens and strengthens the spine.
• It allows blood flow to the head and neck, which will awaken you and stimulate the brain.

DOWNWARD DOG TRANSITION

This can become a move in itself; as you become more experienced, aim to make the move more dynamic.

1 To practise this transition move, lift up and down on your heels to ready yourself for the next move.
2 Push off with your toes and lift your hips as high as you can, bending your knees up towards your chest.
3 If you can, you should hit a balance point before you land your feet between your hands.

THE WARRIOR POSTURES

There are two Warrior positions and they are both great for developing good posture. They work the leg muscles and arm muscles as you reach outwards and upwards, but they also work the torso because the emphasis is on lifting up and out.

You will have already covered this position as part of your Sun Salutation B sequence (see page 63), but doing some further work in this position will strengthen your body further.

WARRIOR 1

You can enter this position from the Downward Dog position by twisting one foot inwards – as in Sun Salutation B (see page 69) – or you can simply jump both feet into a wide position and turn them.

1 Turn the left foot forwards and the right foot inwards to an angle of 45 degrees.
2 Now bend the left knee while keeping the right leg straight and lower into the lunge position. Make sure the left knee isn't pressing forwards of the left foot.
3 Press your groin down towards the floor and reach upwards with your arms, pressing your hands

together as you inhale. Hold this for 5 deep breaths. **4** When you have run though your checklist and have taken 5 breaths along with it, move onto the next posture.

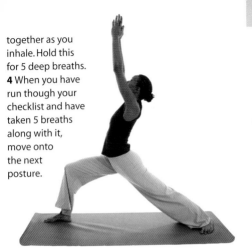

Check

While you are breathing, check the following:
- You are pressing your right foot down all the way round, particularly at the outer edge.
- Your back leg is fully extended and the knee is pulled up.
- You can feel the work in your front thigh – not the knee.
- Check that your bandhas are in place.

WARRIOR 2

1 From Warrior 1, straighten your legs and bring your palms apart.

2 Slowly take your arms out to the sides of your body and bend your front leg again into the lunge.

3 Keep your rib cage and torso facing sideways, and breathe deeply for 5 breaths.

4 Work through the Warrior 1 checklist (see page 97) plus the checklist below.

Check

• Your torso is facing sideways while your arms are reaching out to the ends of the room.
• Direct your gaze over your front arm; feel your chest widening and shoulder blades working.

HALF MOON

This posture is important as it promotes balance.
In yoga, we have to maintain our balance (not just
pass through it) and therefore we may have to
struggle to hold a position – for example, on one foot.
As we struggle to stay upright, we use and strengthen
smaller muscles, which get overlooked in standard
exercises but work together to balance the body.

1 Stand tall with arms
reaching above the head.
2 Slowly start transferring
your balance towards your
left foot. Begin to push your
left hip out to the side also.
3 To balance yourself, bend your
upper torso and arms over to the right.
Taking it further: Once you are
confident in your balance, hold the
stretch as you work on extending
it further by pushing the hips one
way and the upper body the other.
4 Work the stretch for 5 breaths.
5 Lift the arms to bring the body
back to centre, and repeat on
the other side.

THE TRIANGLE

The Triangle (Trikonasana) is a well-known posture. Like most yoga positions, it involves a struggle; this time between the upper and lower body.

1 Start off by jumping your feet wide apart (if this is too difficult, you can step them apart).

2 Pull up on the kneecaps to tighten your thighs. Reach your arms out to the sides, palms facing down.

3 Inhale. Turn your left foot towards the wall, and your right foot at an angle of 45 degrees.

4 With your arms fully extended, reach further with the right arm to pull your body over to the right, exhaling as you do so. Keep this impetus going, so the pull of the right arm pulls your body over to the side.

5 As you lean over, keep your rib cage and upper torso facing sideways and your arms, shoulders and hips in the same vertical plane.

6 The struggle comes as you continue leaning over with your torso facing sideways – there is a tendency to let the rib cage fall forwards to permit a better lean. Do not be tempted to do this or to stick your bottom out behind you. The more you struggle to maintain the alignment, the more heat you will generate and the more stretch you will feel along the left side of your body and in your right hip.

7 If you can, hook your first two fingers under your big toe. If you can't reach this far (without letting your hip go), place your hand on your leg for support.

8 Look upwards towards your outstretched hand, and stay like this for 5 breaths.

9 To return to upright, reach further with your right arm and lift the arm and torso up in one movement.

10 Reverse your feet to perform the posture on the other side, and hold for 5 breaths before coming out of it in the same way.

Note: Try this posture if the one shown opposite is too challenging.

LATERAL ANGLE

This posture (Parsvakonasana) encourages greater flexibility in the hips as you bend low and also gives a superb stretch all down one side of the body.

1 Go into this posture from the jumped-wide position of the feet, as in the Triangle (see page 100).

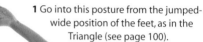

Half Moon

You can practise the Half Moon (see page 99) from this posture, too.

2 Extend both arms out to the sides with your palms facing the floor.
3 Bend your right leg and lean your torso to tip to one side.
4 Place your hand behind your foot if you can, so that your arm pit is just above the knee. Press your knee against your arm with your torso facing forwards. Beginners can place their hand in front of their knee if they find that this is easier.
5 Your upper arm should now be reaching over the side of your body towards the back wall, which is where you are also directing your gaze.
6 Keep the left leg stretched and the full left foot pressing down on the floor.
7 Reach out with your arm and inhale to lift your body back up to centre. Now you can perform the posture on the other side.

TWISTING POSES

In the primary series of Ashtanga Yoga, there are some challenging yet enjoyable twisting postures. When you first attempt the twists, they can seem utterly impossible, but they are not. As you continue to practise, you will start to loosen bits of your body you didn't even know were tight, yet it will feel great!

BOUND KNEE STRETCH

1 Sit on the floor with legs outstretched, then pull your right leg into your body and inhale. Try to get the heel as close to your buttock as you can while keeping your back upright.
2 Now exhale, lean forwards and try to drop your right shoulder in front of your right knee. Press your arm pit against the front of the knee.
3 Wrap your right arm around your right shin and thigh.
4 Bring your left arm back

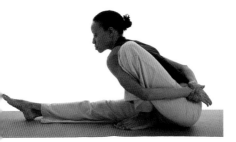

behind you and try to connect the two hands.
Taking it further: Aim to grab your left wrist with your right hand – if this is not possible, however, just hold the fingers.
5 Release yourself from this posture and perform a Sun Salutation before attempting this posture on the other side.

Vinyasa

In between each move in Sun Salutation A until Downward Dog is Vinyasa, a transitional move used to link the movements together and provide flow from one side to another and on to the next move. From Downward Dog, you jump and step through to the position for your next posture.

HALF-BOUND LOTUS

This is another posture that uses the Lotus position (which you have already learnt on page 87) but combines it with the binding. This term refers to the wrapping around of some other part of the body. Binding allows a stretching of certain body parts, particularly helping to loosen hip and shoulder joints that may have stiffened up with age.

1 Start by sitting on the floor with legs outstretched.
2 Now inhale and lift up your right leg, cradling the foot in both hands, and place the back of the foot on the left thigh (this might feel very uncomfortable at first).

3 Try to press the heel of the foot right into the lower abdomen wall. Keep your left thigh facing forwards; don't allow it to fall out to the side.

4 Exhale and reach your right arm behind you and take hold of the big toe of the left foot.

5 Straighten your back and, as you exhale, press your torso forwards, so that your nose is towards your knee. Gaze out towards your toes.

Note: If you can't bind fully, then try holding your right foot with your left hand and wrapping your right arm behind your back and holding onto the left arm. This is a good practice for further binding.

WIDE LEG FORWARD BEND

This posture works on stretching out the backs of the legs, the lower back and hip joints. It also will bring blood to the head, refreshing your brain and invigorating your outlook for the day.

1 Start by jumping (or stepping) your feet wide apart.
2 Contract your thigh muscles to pull up your knees and press the outsides of your feet well into the floor.
3 Take your arms out to the sides and lift your chest.

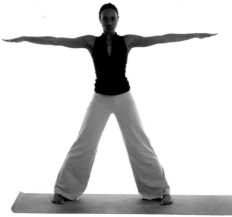

4 Lean back slightly, then tip forwards, directly from the hips to bring your head towards the floor. If you can, use the traction of your hands on the floor to pull your head down to touch it. Remain for 5 breaths.

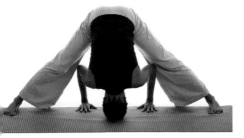

5 Now inhale and lift your head and chest, hands still on the floor.

6 Exhale to place your hands on your hips.

7 Inhale to lift your body up and into a small back arch. Exhale and relax.

Check

While you're breathing, work through your checklist:
- Are your bandhas in place?
- Gaze to the back of the room – is full breath work going on?

VARIATION 1

1 After lifting up, extend your arms out to the sides and place your hands on your hips.
2 Inhale as you arch back and look upwards.
3 Exhale as you fold forwards again, keeping your hands on your hips.
4 Keep your legs tight and bandhas in place. Try to ensure that your coccyx is pointing directly to the ceiling so you are fully folded.
5 The hands on your hips will remind you to engage your abdominal muscle and the pelvic floor (the bandhas on page 44).
6 Remain here for 5 breaths, then come out of the pose as above.

VARIATION 2

1 From wide standing, extend your arms out to the sides.

2 Now link your arms, keeping them straight, behind your back.

3 Lean back into a small arch once again, pushing your hands down behind your back, and then tilt forwards.

4 As you hinge at the hips, lift your hands behind you to extend the stretch with your head going towards the floor. Hold it there for 5 breaths.

5 Inhale and look up to lift your chest, lower your arms and straighten to standing.

THE TREE

The Tree is another balance posture which will build inner strength, better body alignment and great control and co-ordination. It also helps to strengthen ankles and feet. Once again, don't be afraid to struggle to stay balanced throughout your 5 breaths. If you are hopping around too much, come out of the pose and then try again with a fresh breath.

1 Start by standing in the Mountain pose (see page 56), then lift your right leg and cradle it in your hands.
2 Carefully place the sole of your right foot against the inner thigh of the left.
3 Lift both arms up above your head and gaze forwards for 5 breaths. Keep reaching and lifting upwards.
4 Lower your arms and then place the foot, with control, back on the ground.
5 Take one deep breath and repeat on the other side.

THE STRUGGLE

At first you may find that the foot simply slips down the other thigh and won't hold in place, but there are ways to combat this:
• Keep the standing leg pulled up and as strong as possible (don't allow the knee to bend).
• Press the sole of the foot hard against the inner thigh to create a tension that stops the foot slipping.
• Press the right knee and thigh backwards – this also helps keep the foot in place.

TAKING IT FURTHER

Once you have mastered this foot hold you can also try placing the foot in the cross-over position.

1 From standing, lift one leg to cradle and then place the foot across the thigh with the back of the foot against the front of the thigh.
2 Press the bent leg back to create the tension to keep it there.
3 Remain for 5 breaths, then lower and repeat on the other side.

SIDE FORWARD BEND

This posture (Parvottanasana) combines a stretch and a twist, helping to open up the hips, intensely stretch the hamstrings and massage the internal organs. The position of the arms also stretches the chest, shoulders and wrists.

1 Start by jumping (or walking) your legs far apart.
2 Turn your right leg sideways and angle the left foot 45 degrees in the same direction.
3 Turn your body to face the right foot and press your inner thighs together.

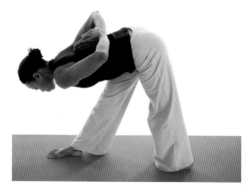

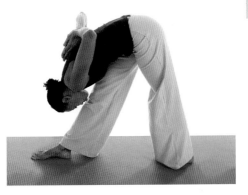

4 Bend your arms behind into a prayer position with fingertips pointing down, then invert the 'V' and bring the fingertips up behind your back. Press the sides of your hand against your upper back to bring the elbow directly out to the side.

5 With your arms in place, tip your body backwards – lift your chest and gaze up and back.

6 Tip forwards to take your nose down to your knee.

7 Press on the outside of your back foot and the inside of your front foot to keep your hips level. You will feel an intense stretch along the front hamstring.

8 Remain and breathe for 5 breaths.

Taking it further: If this position is particularly challenging, remain for 10 breaths in order to allow the muscles to extend further.

9 Inhale as you lift your body up and exhale as you stretch back.

10 Change your feet to the opposite direction and repeat on the other side.

The struggle

If you find it difficult to invert your hands or even press them together in a prayer position, you can simply clasp your elbows and keep your hands in this position for the next phase of the posture.

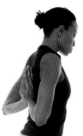

ARM STRETCHES

Here are some additional arm stretches to help you develop flexibility in your shoulders and arms. The first stretch comes from Bikram Yoga.

BIRD OF PARADISE

1 Stand with your feet together and body lifted. Now reach your arms overhead. Clasp your hands, extending the two index fingers.
2 Lock your elbows and press your arms against your ears. Lift up as much as you possibly can. You will feel the stretch in your shoulders.
3 Keep your head lifted to increase the stretch. Breathe for 5 breaths and then release.

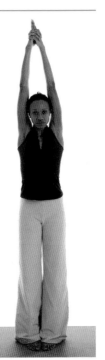

EAGLE ARMS

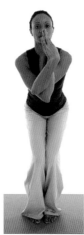

1 Place your right elbow across the your left elbow and wind the forearms around each other, so you can bring the two palms facing each other and together.
2 One arm will be slightly higher than the other but try to press the palms together. Feel the stretch across the front of your shoulders and in the chest area.

3 Remain here for 5 breaths and then release and wrap your arms around the other way.
4 If you can lift one leg and cross it over the supporting knee attempt to wrap it around the other leg, tucking the foot behind the calf. If you lose your balance simply place the foot back on the ground.

OVER-SHOULDER STRETCH

1 Stand tall with your feet touching.
2 Reach one arm over your shoulder and the other arm behind you.
3 Try to grasp both your hands together. If you can't reach, walk your fingertips down your back slowly towards the other hand.
4 Hold for 5 breaths and then repeat with the other arm.

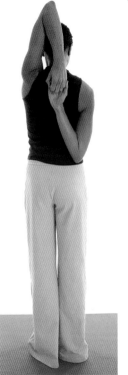

UPPER BODY WORK

Yoga addresses parts of the body that many other exercise regimes leave out. Yet, like other muscles, the eye and neck muscles need work to stay strong and flexible. Here's a short work-out to keep the eyes toned.

EYE EXERCISES

Sit in the Easy Pose (see page 166) or Half Lotus (see page 87). These positions will keep your back straight and allow your shoulders space to drop. Engage the moola bandha (see page 44) to support your back, and rest your wrists on your knees.

1 Look up with your eyes (without moving your head) and back to centre. Repeat 5 times.
2 Look down with your eyes and then back to centre. Repeat 5 times.
3 Look to the far right with your eyes and back to centre. Repeat 5 times.
4 Look to the far left with your eyes and then back to centre. Repeat 5 times.
5 Look diagonally right and return the eyes to centre, then look to diagonal left and return to centre. Repeat alternately 5 times.
6 Take a deep breath and circle your eyes right round

in a circle clockwise, then circle them anticlockwise.
7 Try a 'change of focus' exercise: hold up one finger
in front of your face and focus on it, then switch your
gaze to a wall or horizon far beyond the finger. This
works the long and short focus muscles of the eyes.

Note: Stop immediately if you feel dizzy, and take
some deep breaths.

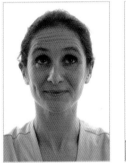 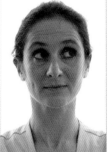

PALMING

1 Rub your hands together to warm them.
2 Cup them and place them over your closed eyes.
Don't press down; simply register the dark and heat,
which will relax your eyes after their hard work.

NECK EXERCISES

The neck is an important area of the body to keep supple. When you warm it up, you send heat around the shoulders and the small muscles in the neck.

1 Start by sitting in the Easy Pose (see page 166) with a straight back.
2 Concentrate on dropping your shoulders down and drop your chin slightly, too, so the back of your neck is lengthened.
3 Inhale and exhale regularly as you move your head.
4 Now tilt your head and press your right ear to your right shoulder.
5 Tilt your head to the other ear and return to centre. Keep your shoulders pulled down; don't allow them to rise up to meet the ear.
6 Keeping your shoulders forward, turn your head and try to look over your shoulder.
7 Turn and look over the other shoulder.
8 Drop your head forward and press your chin to your chest.

Safety

In the position in Step 9 it is very important that you don't throw your head back or tilt it back unsupported. Lift your chin with control and keep your shoulders pressed down – feel as though your head is supported by your neck muscles, not just collapsed backwards.

9 Lift your head up and look upwards.
10 Move your head slowly in a circle clockwise and then anticlockwise. Keep the movement smooth and controlled and don't drop your head back – look up.
11 Return your head to centre and revolve your shoulders round forwards and backwards to finish.

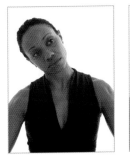
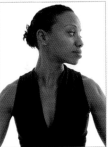

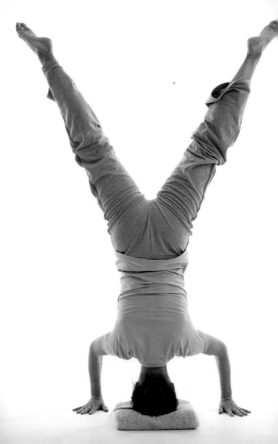

PART SIX

15-minute after-work routine

After work can be a tough time to exercise. You may feel more like collapsing in a chair than motivating yourself to start your yoga routine. However, if you can summon up the energy to do so, you will feel better immediately. The yoga postures in this section will wake up your system, and the blood will flow freely. Many of the postures involve lowering your head below the waist, which is great for refreshing the brain after a stressful day's work.

HEADSTAND VARIATIONS

On page 83 you started working on the Headstand position, but now you can take it further with longer holds and changes of hand positions. Taking your weight on your head may seem strange at first, but the weight is distributed between your arms and head and helps to strengthen your neck.

In order to maintain the balance, a lot of alignment work needs to be done. Your hips need to balance on your rib cage, and the weight is then transferred to your shoulders and from there to your neck and head. Because your body is inverted and balanced on one head as opposed to two evenly spread feet, it needs to be more perfectly aligned, and the small muscles really have to work to achieve this.

Taking it further

You may find some postures challenging but don't be put off. Work on them regularly, using the breath to take you as far into the posture as you can and then come out of it gently. Each time you work a posture, it will get easier to maintain. Yoga is never comfortable – you're always working!

SAFETY

It is considered safer to avoid this position if you suffer from high blood pressure or high cholesterol, or if you are heavily obese or recovering from any form of eye surgery.

Falling

Many people are afraid of falling from a headstand. Try to practise this position near a wall or on a bed initially, unless you have someone to assist you. The safest way to come out of a headstand if you lose control is to try and round your back and roll out of it. You might find yourself arching over with your feet hitting the ground.

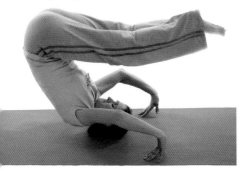

FULL HEADSTAND BALANCE

1 Place your arms in the triangular position with your fingers clasped. Place your head between your hands and lift your hips by straightening your legs.
2 Walk your feet in towards your head to tip the balance of your hips; then you can start to lever your feet off the ground.
3 When you feel this shift in balance, keep lifting your legs slowly.
4 Inhale and lift your legs to vertical. Stay in the full headstand for 5 breaths.
5 To lower yourself, bring your legs down to the horizontal position, then lower, with control, to the floor.

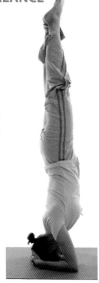

Safety

Attempt this move the first few times with someone present to help support you or against a wall.

HEADSTAND WITH HALFWAY HOLD

1 Perform the headstand and hold for 10 breaths (if you can do so).
2 Slowly lower your legs with control, but this time only halfway and hold them there for 5 breaths.
3 Lower to the ground with control.

THE SCORPION

With your new-found confidence in movement, strength and alignment, you can attempt this. The weight in a Scorpion stand is taken by your shoulders and chest muscles, and there are different methods of getting into the posture.

1 Place your forearms on the mat; spread your hands flat and spread your fingers for balance.
2 Walk your feet in slightly to lift your hips above your body, then kick your legs into the air. It is safer to kick robustly as your body will rise up; if you kick half-heartedly you may come down hard on your toes.
3 If you fall, bend one leg quickly; lower the other. If you over-balance the other way, your foot will hit the wall.
4 Once you hit the position, try to keep your body as straight as possible and don't allow your back to arch too far.
5 Take 5 breaths, then lower with control.

SCORPION SHOULDER STRETCH

If you don't feel up to attempting the Scorpion yet,
work on the Shoulder Stretch posture. If you have
tight shoulders, you may find the Scorpion difficult,
so practising this first will certainly help.

1 Kneel on the mat and place your arms and hands
flat on the floor.
2 Now walk your feet in and lift your hips up until
you feel them over your shoulders or very near.
3 Hold this position and feel the stretch (and the
work) in the shoulder area. Hold for 5 breaths.
4 Lift up onto your toes and then lower your
heels back down to the floor; do this 3 times.
5 Bend your knees
to come out of
the stretch.

THE LOCUST

This is another posture that requires the ability to kick up into the air and rely on your body to keep you straight and safe. When you are in a full lift, it builds strength in your upper and lower back and hamstrings. The initial lift of the legs builds strength in the buttocks and lower back.

1 Lie on the floor on your front, resting your chin on the floor with your neck straight and gaze forward.
2 Lift your hips slightly off the floor and tuck your

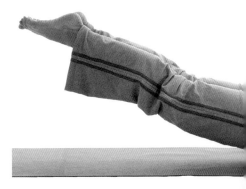

arms underneath your body with your elbows close together. The back of your hands should be flat on the mat and your arms straight.

3 You are aiming to lift your legs, but when you start this may feel impossible! However, as you keep practising, it becomes easier.

4 Press the backs of your arms into the floor and, exhaling, lift one leg off the floor until it is raised behind you, pointing outward and as straight as possible with the toes pointed.

5 Lower your leg and repeat with the other leg. If you can't lift it very high to begin with, don't worry – just keep working at it.

6 Lower the second leg, then take a deep breath.

7 Now try to lift both legs and keep them up in the air for 5 breaths. If you need to lower them after less than 5 breaths, that's okay – just enter the position again to complete the 5 breaths.

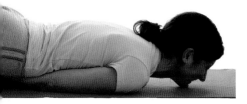

THE BOW

There are many kinds of back bending postures in yoga to strengthen and mobilize the back of the body. The back gets a real flex in this posture in a plane that everyday movement doesn't normally take us to. The back arching of the central axis is actually very beneficial for the spine. It is thought that resting on the abdominal area aids digestion, too. The Bow is one of the easiest back-bend postures in yoga.

1 Lie on your stomach and then bend your legs up behind you.
2 Inhale and grab your ankles with your hands.
3 Exhale and try to lift your chest and thighs off the floor. You will feel tension between the pulling on your arms and your legs, but keep arching as much as you can.
4 Breathe for 5 breaths, then slowly release the arch and then the hold on your ankles.

TAKING IT FURTHER

When you have mastered the Bow, you can have a go at moving within the posture – not across the room but by rocking from end to end.

1 Lift your feet up into the Bow posture.

2 Keeping hold of your feet, aim to rock slightly from head to feet.

Note: You can also try rocking onto the side of your body and back up again.

THE COBRA

This is another great posture for the back: it flexes the spine, keeps the back of the body supple and encourages the back to move in all directions.

1 Lie on the floor with your head resting on the floor and arms by your sides.
2 Bring your palms up to rest next to your shoulders with elbows resting on the floor.
3 Exhale and press on your arms to lift your head and shoulders off the floor.

4 Gently try to straighten your arms and extend the arch, but only straighten your arms all the way if you can keep your hips on the floor – don't lift your hips up as this stops the arch.
5 Hold this posture for 5 breaths, then release down.

THE STRUGGLE

Your objective in the Cobra is to keep your hip bones in contact with the floor yet lift your chest as high and as far back as you can. In order to do this, you will need to really tighten your buttock muscles and use the muscles along the back bone (the erector spine) to lift and maintain the arch. You will feel your chest widening as you arch and also work happening in your arms.

FORWARD SEATED BEND

This is a great counter posture to all the previous spine flexing ones, such as the Cobra, Bow and Locust. A counter posture is one that works the body in the opposite way to the previous pose, thereby relieving and flexing it in a different direction at the same time.

The folding nature of this posture stretches out the back of the body – stretching the hamstrings and the lower and upper back. It also massages the internal organs as you compress forward.

1 Sit up straight with your hands by your hips.
2 Lean forwards as you exhale and link your fingers around your big toes. Beginners can hold onto

their ankles if they cannot reach their toes.

3 Inhale and lift upwards in this position, trying to straighten your back and drop your shoulders.

4 Exhale and lean further forwards. Try to rest your body on top of your legs and bring your nose to your knees. Your arms should be relaxed on the floor if possible.

5 Remain here for 5 breaths.

TAKING IT FURTHER

As you take your 5 deep breaths, let the exhale lower you further onto your knees. Try to keep your back relatively straight and your neck extended. If, to begin with, your head is far away from your knees, don't worry; simply work with the breath to slowly inch closer. As you repeat this posture over the weeks and months, you will be amazed at how much flexibility you gain.

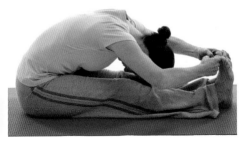

THE PLANK

Now that you have flexed your spine both backwards and forwards you are going to work on keeping it perfectly straight. This posture is less about flexibility and more about strength. This is the beauty of yoga; it marries flexibility work perfectly with strength work, giving you the best combination of suppleness and endurance to keep your body capable of virtually any movement for as many years as you keep practising. Yoga moves performed by people in their eighties will keep them as supple as people in their forties.

This posture is part of the Sun Salutation sequence, so you will have attempted it already, but this 15-minute after-work session will give you another opportunity to perfect it even further.

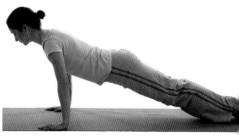

1 To come into this posture (without the previous build up of the Sun Salutation), lie on your stomach and rest your chin on the mat.

2 Place your hands on the mat next to your chest and tuck your toes under to push them against the mat.

3 Exhale and, while pushing on your hands and gripping with your toes, lift your body off the floor. Your hips, thighs, chest and nose should all be just off the floor.

4 Lift your head to gaze forwards. Remain like this for 5 breaths.

TAKING IT FURTHER

Pushing up into this position may seem really tough (tougher than lowering yourself into it as you do in the Sun Salutation), but this is what will build your muscular endurance. Try to hold the position without lifting or sinking the mid-section of your body.

Make it easier

If, initially, you cannot maintain the hold for a full 5 breaths, you can rest your body by dropping your knees on to the floor and resting briefly. Then straighten the knees off the floor and tighten back into the position.

THE BOAT

This posture also works on developing muscular endurance rather than flexibility, although it does require some mobility (which you should have by now) in the back of your legs. It also requires – and promotes – strength in the mid-section of the body, and uses the abdominal muscles and hip flexor muscles to maintain the shape. After practising this posture regularly, you will notice increased strength and control in your whole middle section.

1 Sit on the floor with your legs and back straight.
2 Now draw up your knees, so that just the toes are touching the floor.
3 At the same time, roll back on your hips slightly, so that your weight is back.

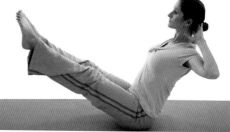

4 Exhale and extend your legs out.

5 When you feel balanced, take your arms behind your head and flex your feet – toes towards the face.

6 Hold for 5 breaths.

7 Bend your legs back in to come out of the pose. Beginners can tip back and leave their hands on the floor and just work on raising their legs.

TAKING IT FURTHER

Think about using your bandhas (see page 44) to hold the position. Struggle to keep your back from rounding, and try to press your upper thighs against your lower stomach. To build strength in this area, this posture is often repeated up to 5 times. Move into the posture, hold for 5 breaths, release your legs and place them in the Easy Pose. Make one inhale and exhale before moving back into the Boat. Repeat 5 times.

Check

While you are holding, work through the following:
• Are the bandhas (see page 44) in place?
• Are you struggling to keep the tops of your thighs pressing towards your lower stomach?
• Are you struggling to keep your back as straight as possible?

BOAT WITH OARS

This posture is a further development of the previous pose. In this posture, rather than balancing your legs by leaning back and placing your hands behind you, your arms are reaching forwards, which makes the balance more challenging.

1 Start by sitting on the floor (as with the previous pose) with your toes just touching.
2 Now lean back and extend your legs, at the same time extending your arms forwards as if they were a pair of oars steering your very own boat.
3 Hold this posture for 5 breaths.

Transitional movement

Between each repetition of this pose, you can also try a form of Vinyasa, which means a linking sequence between postures.

1 Coming out of the pose, keeping your legs raised, cross them in front of you.

2 Place your hands on the floor to lift your bottom and legs entirely off the floor.

3 Your body is now suspended by your hands and arms, supported by the lift of your bandhas.

4 Hold just briefly and then lower your body to the floor to press back into a second repetition of the posture (opposite).

THE ROD

Coming out of the previous Boat postures for the last time, you can lower your legs and move into this posture (Dandasana), which you can use every day. Every time you sit on the floor, make use of the principles learned and practised here to keep your spine straight and supported and your body lifted.

Even when sitting down or working, you can use the principles from this posture to keep your everyday alignment perfect. A lifted upper torso allows more room for the stomach and its contents and the lungs to do their work. It keeps the spine straight and healthy, rather than slumped forward and cramped. Practise this posture every day to help prevent backache.

1 Lower your legs from the previous Boat posture straight onto the floor.

2 Press your hands down into the floor by your hips.

3 Hold this position for 5 breaths.

4 While you hold, try to think about lifting up through the top of your head, so that you feel your spine elongating. Drop your chin slightly to elongate the back of your neck, and feel the energy press across your chest, so it widens and the shoulder blades draw back.

5 Press your legs together and pull up on your thighs and pull back your feet.

6 Pull up on your bandhas.

WORKING A POSE

As with all the yoga postures, the Rod perfectly illustrates one of the key concepts of yoga – that of constantly working a pose. Whilst an outsider looking at someone in this position might assume that they are merely resting, a practising yogi will understand that even the simplest poses are opportunities to tone, challenge and work the muscles throughout every breath of the pose.

You can work on pulling the shoulder blades down, pulling up on the knees and working the feet back without looking as though you are doing anything.

STANDING FORWARD BEND

Having worked the previous posture, you will have readied your legs for some further stretching. Now you can come to standing for a further leg stretch. This posture (Uttanasana) will stretch out the back of your body and will stimulate the inner organs as you fold. It will also bring blood to your head and scalp. You have already used this posture in the Sun Salutations, but this is a chance to work it further.

1 Begin as if you are coming from a Sun Salutation and reach your arms upwards, drawing your body up as tall as it will go.

2 Reach your arms forwards and fold your body over and place your hands on the floor. If you can't do this, simply place your hands further up your legs – for instance, on the shins or even the knees.

3 Try to keep your legs as straight as possible and pull your thighs up – bend your knees if necessary to keep the fold.

4 In the fold, try to flatten your back further and struggle to press your stomach against your thighs.

5 Use the grip of your hands on the floor (or legs) to pull your head in further.

6 As you take your 5 slow breaths, try to imagine that you are breathing oxygen into the backs of your legs

to relieve the intense stretch in this area.
7 Come out of the position by stretching your arms forwards to lift your upper torso back up.

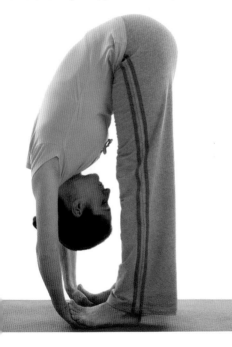

THE HERO

This posture is unique; you will not come across it in any other form of exercise. It will stretch out the backs of your feet and ankles, your knees and hips.

1 Start by kneeling on your legs with a straight back, and rest your hands on your knees.
2 Stay here for several breaths and check that this is relatively comfortable. If so, progress to the next stage.

3 Take your feet about 45cm (18in) apart and try to rest your buttocks on the floor. To do this, you may need to pull your calves out from under your thighs.
4 Keep your back straight, your knees together and your feet parallel to your thighs.
5 Rest here for 5 breaths.

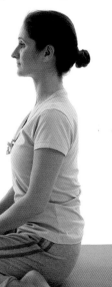

THE STRUGGLE

This posture is less of a struggle and is more about letting go. Try to allow your muscles and ligaments to release, so that you can sink into this position. At first it may seem very uncomfortable on your hips and feet, but the more you gently hold this position – and breathe – the easier it will become. What will happen is that your hips will open up as will your knee joints and thigh muscles, making your whole lower body much more flexible.

TAKING IT FURTHER

If you can achieve this posture successfully, then you can try extending one leg out in front of you. This is good preparation for the yoga posture Tiryan Mukhaikapada Paschimottanasana (not shown in this book).

THE COBBLER

This posture stretches the body yet strengthens it at the same time. It looks deceptively simply but, as with all yoga positions, it incorporates the struggle of opposing forces of the body.

1 Sit with legs apart and back straight.
2 Bend your legs, so that your feet are touching.
3 Straighten your back.
4 Gently try to press your knees towards the floor. When you get them to the floor, check that your spine is straight and cup your feet with your hands.
5 Hold this position for 5 breaths.

THE STRUGGLE

The difficulty for most people who are performing the Cobbler posture will be getting their knees to hit the floor. To get anywhere near, you will have to press your thighs actively while lifting out of the lower back to avoid curving. Press your shoulder blades together and roll your shoulders back to open out your chest.

PREPARATION WORK

If you have trouble with this position and cannot stay upright and/or get your knees to fall outwards at all, then you may need to do some preparation work to help you, as outlined below.

1 Sit with your legs bent and feet touching, but lean back on your hands to support your back.
2 Gently rock your legs from side to side, so that the knee on one side touches the floor, and then rock to the other side to touch the other knee down. This a non-threatening way of getting your hips used to the idea of expanding a little.
3 When this feels comfortable, you can try to push yourself more upright and perform the same rock.
4 From here, you can progress to the Cobbler pose (see page 153).

SEATED ANGLE

This posture (Upavista konasana) will also open your hips and stretch your legs and feet but in a totally different way to the Cobbler (see page 153).

1 Start by sitting on the floor with your back straight and legs flat out in front of you.
2 Open your legs as wide as you can.
3 Draw up the height through your spine and lift.
4 Slowly try to lean forwards, placing your hands in front of you to minimize the risk of injury.
5 Try to keep your feet turned up to the ceiling as you press your upper body forward towards the mat. If you can get far enough forwards, hold your instep with your hands.
6 Hold here for 5 breaths. You will be stretching the inner thigh muscles as you lean forwards. Don't worry if you cannot get your chest to the floor – just lean forwards and breathe.

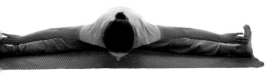

THE STRUGGLE

This is in the hip joints and the inner thighs. These are the areas where you will feel the muscles resisting and where you have to slowly work on the stretch.

Taking it further

• Use your hands to grip the mat and inch your body forwards to progress the stretch.
• For each new forward position you reach, stay in it and breathe for up to 10 breaths. Over time, this will loosen the muscles and allow you to press forwards further and further.

Make progress fast

Like all postures in yoga, the more frequently you practise (preferably every day), the faster you will progress and the more satisfying your practice will be. Even if you just spend 15 minutes (which is, after all, what this book is all about) each day, you will start to notice small but significant improvements in all areas of your flexibility and suppleness. Try to make your yoga practice part of your regular routine. Even if you don't have much time and cannot manage 15 minutes, anything is better than nothing, so keep it regular.

HIP TWIST

Twists are great for the spine, mobilizing the vertebrae, bringing fresh blood to the area and toning the back muscles. Although this posture (Bharadvajasana) looks like a relatively simple twist, it is a killer, particularly if you have tight shoulders. Practise diligently!

1 Start by kneeling on both knees. Sit tall and breathe deeply.
2 Shift your buttocks to one side, so your feet are next to your left hip. Aim to rest both buttocks on the floor.
3 Start the twist in the lower body, turning, so you can place your left hand on your right knee.

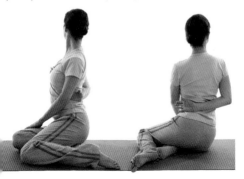

4 Keep that arm firmly placed as you twist further and reach behind with your right arm to grab your left elbow. **5** Hold the position for 5 breaths, breathing deeper into the twist with each breath.

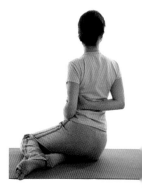

BEGINNERS

Initially, you may find it easier to approach this stretch slightly differently. After positioning your legs and lengthening your spine, reach behind with your right arm and take hold of the left, then begin the twist. This will allow you to stretch your shoulders (with the left arm as anchor) to get into the twist.

Tightness in the body

Yoga postures are excellent for stretching more than one area of the body. Wherever you feel the most resistance is the area, you are most tight – this is excellent body information to possess.

DOUBLE TWIST

This posture (Gomukhasana) stretches the hip joints, shoulder joints and chest muscles at the same time. Lift up throughout all the seated poses and use the breath to settle more comfortably into each pose.

1 Sit on the floor with one leg bent, knee facing forward and the other leg bent across the top, one knee on top of the other.
2 Lift up through your torso and exhale as you take one arm over the top of your shoulder.
3 Reach the other arm behind your back; try to clasp your hand behind.
4 Remain here for 5 breaths.

THE STRUGGLE

As you breathe, try to bring your hands closer together by extending your shoulder joints. Work your hands against each other to grip higher up the top hand. Work your legs as well and try to rest your

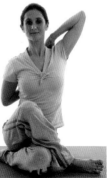

knees flat on top of each other. You will feel this in your hips as you work. You will also feel your chest being stretched wide.

• Be careful not to force your knees into position – use the breath.

• Release your legs and arms to repeat the posture on the other side.

TAKING IT FURTHER

For an extra limber in your arms, lean your hands against a wall and walk your feet backwards until your torso is parallel to the floor. In this position, gently press your chest towards the floor and feel the stretch in your shoulder joints. Gently move to and fro to work the stretch on the shoulders a little deeper.

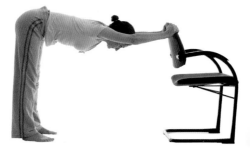

BOUND KNEE STRETCH

This pose (Marichyasana) is a challenging twist but it is a great way of stimulating the internal organs. It also stretches out the arms and shoulders once again.

1 Sit on the floor and draw your right leg up so that your heel is next to your sitting bone.
2 The outside of your right foot should be in line with the outer edge of your hip. Your right foot should not touch your left inner thigh.
3 Exhale and lean forwards, and drop your right shoulder in front of your knee.
4 Keep your right palm facing away from your body. Wrap your arm round your knee.
5 Take your left arm behind you; let your right hand grab on to it.
6 Look over your shoulder away from your bent leg.
7 Remain in this position for 5 breaths.

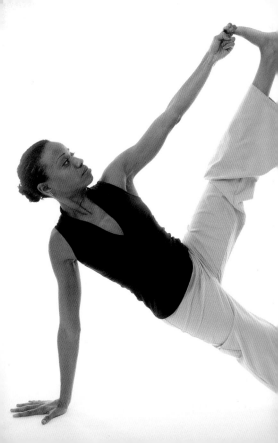

PART SEVEN

15-minute bedtime routine

Doing some work with your body before bedtime can be beneficial, but being too active can be counter-productive as it may be difficult to wind down and sleep. This is why it's not a good idea to exercise late into the evening. However, sitting down watching television is equally bad as it can lead to stiff muscles or worse. Relax your body by using the following yoga postures.

THE CAT

This may be a familiar posture as it has infiltrated many exercise regimes. It is a great way of mobilizing a stiff back and arching the spine both up and down as well as stimulating the inner organs.

1 Start on all-fours and distribute your weight equally across your hands and knees.
2 Exhale and arch your back upwards (like an angry cat).
3 Drop your head down.
4 Pull up through the centre of your back as if you are trying to stick your spine on the ceiling.
5 Pull up on your abdominal muscles to help the arch and stimulate the inner organs.
6 Maintain this posture for 5 breaths.

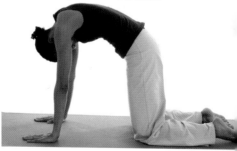

7 Now release the arch and this time press your spine down past neutral until you are arching your stomach down towards the floor. You will feel your back flex and your shoulder blades pull back.

8 Hold this position for just 2 breaths and then arch upwards again. Repeat 2–3 times.

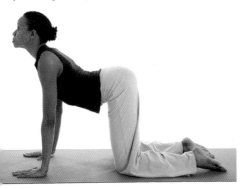

NEUTRAL SPINE

This is where the pelvis is tilted neither backwards nor forwards. Lie on the floor with your knees bent and feet flat. There should be a small gap under your lower back but not a large one. Your pelvis should not be tilted so far up that your back is flat on the ground.

EASY POSE

This yoga posture is worth using all the time – not just when you're doing a yoga session! It's a good way to support your back when sitting as it is not easy to slouch in this position. It also allows the upper body to be aligned correctly and the neck and head to be held comfortably. Keeping your legs tucked underneath you is actually good for blood flow (as long as you don't stay there too long) rather than the blood flowing down to the lower legs all the time.

1 Sit with your legs crossed on the floor.
2 Lift your back straight and allow your shoulders to

Yoga promotes flexibility

Flexibility is a form of exercise in itself that many people overlook. Stretching your muscles not only returns them to their original length after contractions but also stimulates them together with the bones they pull on. Stretching can iron out kinks or air locks in the muscles and joints that may have built up over the day, so when you stretch and mobilize in the evening you are reviving and relaxing your body ready for sleep.

drop and the top of your head to feel as if it is lifting towards the ceiling.

3 Relax your legs and feel the weight of the thighs fall into the mat.

4 Stretch your spine out by lifting your arms and clasping your hands together, pressing the palms up to the ceiling. Feel the stretch along the outsides of the upper arms and forearms.

WHEN TO USE THE EASY POSE

Try sitting in the Easy Pose on the floor, rather than a sofa, when you are watching TV. You can also try it sitting on a wide chair when listening to music. However, it may not go down so well at the office!

THE SWAN

This stretches out and relieves tension in the lower back and shoulders and brings blood to the head.

1 Kneel with your bottom on your knees. Keep your body tall and upright and shoulders pulled down.
2 Lean forwards and come onto all-fours with your weight on your hands also.
3 Exhale. Slide your hands forwards, extending your shoulders and pressing your arm pits towards the floor.

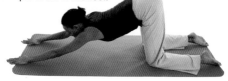

4 Keep pressing until your forehead is on the mat and your arms are extended beyond your head. Your legs are at right angles.

5 Hold this position for 5 breaths.
6 Come back to kneeling to recover.

ADDITIONAL POSE

You can also transfer this position to a standing one and place your hands against a wall or on a barre.

1 Press your hands against the wall or lay them on a solid table or barre. Now keeping the hands in contact with the barre/wall , walk the feet back until your arms are straight out above your head. Your arm pits and face are facing the floor. Hold for 5 breaths as you feel the stretch along the back and shoulders. You will also feel the stretch up the back of the legs.
2 Keep the abdomen and the lower back lifted but press down gently on the shoulders.

Taking it further

The pose to the left is a further stretch for the back and shoulders. You will often see cats doing this.
1 Press the arm pits towards the floor while keeping your backside lifted.
2 Push your weight slightly forward to lower your chin towards the floor.

CHILD POSE

You can extend the previous position (the Swan) even further and take it into what is known as the Child Pose. This is a total relaxation pose and is great for relieving the lower back.

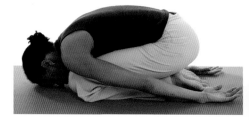

1 Start on all-fours with equal weight on your hands and knees.
2 From this position, slide your hands forwards and lower your bottom towards your feet.
3 Come to rest with your bottom sat fully on your feet and your head resting on the mat with your arms extended.
4 Now move your arms down beside your hips and rest them on the mat, palms facing upwards.
5 Breathe and rest for 5 breaths.

6 Move your hands and place them over your feet.
7 Breathe for another 5 breaths.

TAKING IT FURTHER

If you have a friend or partner available, then ask
them – while you are still in this position – to place
a little of their weight on your lower back to extend
the stretch even further. This will feel very restful and
may send you to sleep!

The weight placed by your partner on the bottom
of your spine lifts the weight off the upper back. This
allows the muscles along
the back to unclench,
and you will experience
a relaxing feeling of
well-being.

LYING TWIST

Once you release into it, you will find that this yoga posture is very relaxing, whilst stretching you out at the same time. The movement into the posture itself tones the sides of your torso.

1 Start off by lying on the floor with your legs straight and your arms stretched out to the sides, palms facing upwards.
2 Bend your legs in and then lift them up towards the ceiling.
3 Slowly, and with control, lower your legs over to one side. As you do so, contract the muscles of your torso to prevent your legs from falling with gravity. Your upper body should remain flat on the ground.
4 When your legs are resting on the floor, breathe for 5 breaths. Your feet should be near your outstretched hand, and your head should be looking across at your opposite hand.
5 Press your shoulders and shoulder blades towards the floor and keep your neck relaxed.
6 From one side, bring your legs to vertical. To do this, inhale, tighten your abdominals and use your bandhas to lift your legs.
7 In the vertical position, breathe for 5 breaths.
8 Lower the legs to the other side in the same way.

ALTERNATIVE VERSION

1 Start with your legs bent and feet on the floor.
2 Tip your knees all the way to one side (with control), keeping your feet in contact with the floor.
3 Now rest for 5 breaths with your head looking the other way.
4 Bring your knees to vertical and then over to the other side.
5 With your knees bent, the lifting to vertical will be easier and you will feel a slightly different stretch on the back.

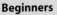

Beginners

Initially you may need to lift first one leg (the one on top), then the other, to propel the knees to vertical.

SUPINE LEG RAISE

The following four postures involve some serious stretching, along with relaxation, so don't forget to use the breath to both relax and flex.

This first posture is all about extending flexibility in your hips and the backs of your legs. This will help you in all your movements in everyday life.

1 Start by lying on the floor with both your arms and legs flat on the floor.
2 Exhale and lift your right leg up to meet your outstretched arm, linking your fingers around your big toes.
3 Keeping your left hip pressed into the floor, exhale and try to bring your leg closer towards your nose.
4 Breathe for 5 breaths whilst working to bring your leg closer with each exhalation.

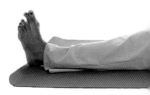

THE STRUGGLE

You must work to keep your knee pulled up and your leg as straight as possible while encouraging your leg down towards your nose. This will feel uncomfortable and will build heat to allow a stretch to occur.

• After 5 breaths, slowly lower your leg and exhale to lift the other leg up.
• If holding onto the toe is not possible, bend your leg to grab hold of the toe. Pull the bent leg towards you in the same way. Remain for 5 breaths, straightening the leg as much as you can.
• Repeat on the other leg.

SUPINE SIDE LEG RAISE

This posture follows on perfectly from the previous one. After you have finished working on the Supine Leg Raises (see page 174) you can roll onto one side and work on this posture (Anantasana).

1 Roll onto your left side and bend your arm up to support your head. This will stabilize your body as you exhale and lift your leg.
2 Grab your big toe with your fingers and, exhaling, pull

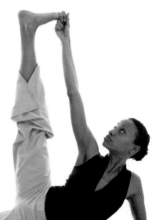

your leg up towards your ear. Feel the stretch and resistance in your inner thigh and hip.

3 Work for 5 breaths at inching the leg closer.

4 Slowly lower your leg, then roll onto the other side to repeat on the other leg.

ALTERNATIVE POSTURE

You can also access this posture without turning onto your side. Simply lay flat (as in the previous posture) and from the Supine Leg Raise lift, inhale, exhale and then pull your leg over to the side, so that you are stretching the side of the inner leg this way. This alternative posture is a more stable position for extending the stretch.

UPWARD FACING BOW

This is a great posture for stretching the abdominals and the whole front of the body along with flexing the spine in a direction that is normally neglected. The posture calls for flexibility and mobility in the shoulders and chest as well as working the muscles in the buttocks and thighs, so it's a tough one.

1 Start by lying on your back on the mat with your legs bent and feet on the floor.
2 Place your palms on the ground next to your ears.
3 Push up with your arms and legs to lift your body off the floor and thrust your abdomen high up in the air.
4 Use your bandhas to help you lift and try to press your arms straight.
5 Try to walk your feet in towards your head a little, so you will have better purchase to press with your legs.
6 Stay and struggle for 5 breaths. The gaze is down towards the mat.

THE STRUGGLE

You're trying to get your shoulders above your hands and to eventually straighten your legs; this would be the perfect Upward Facing Bow posture. You must press with your legs and arms and arch your torso.

• After 5 breaths, lower your head to the floor but keep your legs tensed and working.
• Recover in this position for 3 breaths and then push up into the Bow position for another 5 breaths. Repeat 3 times.

RECOVERY

To recover after this posture, lie on the floor and hug your knees into your chest; breathe slowly and deeply. If you feel this posture is too challenging, ignore it and practise the Bridge (see page 180).

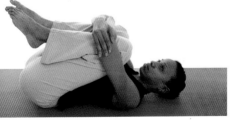

THE BRIDGE

This posture is a gentler way of arching your back and will build strength in the legs and buttock muscles to help support this position and the previous posture.

1 Start by lying on the floor with your legs bent and hands flat on the floor.
2 Exhale and lift your hips up towards the ceiling.
3 Keep your neck straight and your gaze towards the ceiling.
4 Inhale and press your weight slightly towards your head as you arch your back further.
5 Exhale and lift your hands to place them underneath your rib cage to support the posture.
6 Breathe for 5 long breaths.
7 Slowly lower your upper body to finish.

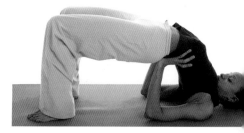

TAKING IT FURTHER

If you are more experienced at yoga, you can enter this posture from the Shoulder Stand.

1 From the Shoulder Stand posture, press your legs strongly upwards.
2 Tip your legs back towards your head, then arch your body to drop your legs towards the floor.
3 Press your hands into your back.
4 Drop your legs to the floor.

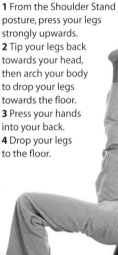

RELAXING AFTER YOGA

It has always been an important part of yoga work that you follow the postures with a period of stillness. The Corpse is the position in which this is done.

THE CORPSE

The Corpse position has been described earlier (see page 77) and it is a simple pose. Just check that your body is positioned squarely on the floor with your legs open and arms slightly out to the sides.

The struggle

There is no need to struggle in the Corpse posture – it is meant for relaxation – but you can use this time profitably to notice some important facts.

FEELING DISCOMFORT

As you lie still after the postures, you may notice some discomfort in your body: you may feel your shoulders aching or your rib cage smarting, or even your hips may be painful. It is important to note where you feel the discomfort, as this will tell you which parts of your body have been put under most stress. In the postures, you have been stretching and strengthening all the body areas and when you come to rest you will be aware of some discomfort. Don't be discouraged; your body is just making readjustments and realignments with its newly stretched muscles and ligaments. As you continue to practise yoga, you will notice this discomfort in every Corpse position you do, but you may find that different areas are releasing, readjusting and realigning as your body changes.

TAKE STOCK

Don't be tempted to skip the Corpse posture – it is during this time that your body takes stock of what you have just put it through. You will notice in your daily life greater flexibility in your body, additional fluidity in your movements and more control and balance in everything you do.

GO MENTAL

While you are lying quietly in the Corpse position, you can use this time to exercise a different part of your system – your brain! Do some meditation or at least some mind control (see page 46). Don't allow yourself to fall asleep. You probably will not feel like it at this time anyway, because your blood will be racing and your body will be heated from the hard work you have done. Instead, use this time to focus on what your body is feeling or simply rein your attention in (see overleaf).

Stay focused

• Find a mark on the ceiling – anything that you can make out – on which to focus and try and keep your attention on it. Study the crack in the paintwork, the odd shape of a pattern or a discolouration of the wallpaper – anything that keeps your mind from wandering. Stay focused on this while you wait for your body aches to ebb away.

• When your body is comfortable is when you are ready to come out of the Corpse posture.

TAKING IT FURTHER

While you are in the Corpse posture, you can also try practising some body mapping. This is just a way of being more aware of your body.

1 Lie on the floor on your back and rest your limbs.
2 Feel the weight of your head on the floor and think about the muscles in your neck and how they feel now you have done your work-out.
3 Think about your shoulders and whether they are lifted off the floor or falling towards the ground. Think about whether they feel relaxed or more stretched out. Notice where the readjustments are.
4 Think about your middle back and your rib cage and which part of the back of your rib cage is

touching the ground. Does any specific part feel more released now?

5 Think about the whole of the length of your spine. Register any tension and make a note of where your body may be changing. Notice where your spine touches the floor and where it is lifted off the ground. Notice if there any areas of discomfort or tension.

6 Think about your buttocks and upper thighs. Notice where they press into the floor and where they do not touch. Is there equal weight on both sides of your pelvis?

7 Think about your calves and feet. Register any tension or discomfort.

8 Notice, but don't try to change, any discomfort; add it to your body knowledge and learn from it.

Note: Performing this kind of body stock take regularly will make you more aware of your body and help you to control and prevent any injuries.

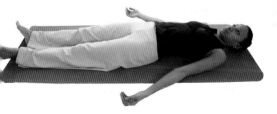

TAKING IT FURTHER

You have now come to understand the basics of yoga practice and how it can improve not only your body but also your mind and your outlook.

This book has focused on how just 15 minutes every day can make a difference and implant a practice mentality. It is your turn, however, to take it further. As you get stronger and your practice becomes more instinctive, you can start to lengthen your sessions. A longer session will allow you to cover more postures and therefore practise more on each body part.

All the yoga systems, including Ashtanga, Iyengar and Sivananda, have a full hour or more regime that is the recommended practice, so try and build up the length of practice slowly.

BOOKS TO CONTINUE YOUR PRACTICE

There are many specialist yoga books that can be recommended to complement this one should you wish to find out more about the subject, but you should experiment with different styles of yoga to see which one suits you best. Here are some useful titles for you to look at.

Bender-Birch, Beryl, *Power Yoga* (Prion Books)
Bender-Birch, Beryl, *Beyond Power Yoga* (Simon & Schuster)
Collins, *Need to know? Yoga* (HarperCollins)
Iyengar, B.K.S., *Light on Yoga* (HarperCollins)
Sivandra Yoga Centre, *The New Book of Yoga* (Ebury Press)
Swenson, David, *Ashtanga Practice Manual* (Ashtanga Yoga Productions)

CLASSES

Don't forget that classes can add to your home practice and can help you to extend the length of your practice with new postures. A good teacher will also make adjustments and observations that you cannot make yourself – so class attendance, at least once in a while, is a good idea.

PERSONAL TRAINING

If you can find yourself a personal yoga teacher to visit your home and observe your practice from time to time, it will be very beneficial. Working one-on-one, a good trainer can really extend your practice and push you in the areas that you wish to develop and are specific to you. You can find a trainer in the UK by logging on to www.iapf.co.uk.

CHILDREN AND PREGNANCY

Young yoga is gaining popularity and can prove very beneficial to teens and even younger children. They can learn balance, body awareness and strength from doing yoga moves. It is a paced and calm way of moving that even children, with their busy out-of-school schedules, can enjoy as a relaxation session away from the frenetic pace of the playground. Very young children can benefit from the experience of yoga moves, with postures being adapted for groups and the posture names altered to reflect the natural world of birds, animals or insects. See the websites (opposite) for information on classes.

During pregnancy, yoga can calm and prepare the mother to be. Yoga postures need to be adapted for pregnancy, to take account of the growing foetus, so consult a qualified yoga teacher to alter your programme. The meditation, breathing and deep relaxation skills can help foster a calm and enjoyable pregnancy, whilst the mastering of the locks and general strengthening of the entire body will help with the arduous task of labour. Postnatally you can gradually rebuild strength and suppleness with carefully chosen yoga work. Consult a qualified yoga teacher with direct experience of yoga for pregnancy.

FIND OUT MORE

British Wheel of Yoga
25 Jermyn Street,
Sleaford,
Lincolnshire NG34 7RU
Tel: 01529 306851
Fax: 01529 303233

**Ashtanga Yoga
Research Institute**
For all Ashtanga
related information
email:ashtangafilm@hot
mail.com

Sivananda style Yoga
www.Sivananda.org

General information
www.healthandyoga.com

Yoga for beginners
www.healthandyoga.com

Yoga in pregnancy
www.healthandyoga.com

Yoga for children
www.relaxkids.com
www.yogabugs.com

Yoga for men
For information and
the benefits:
www.abc-of-yoga.com

YOGA Magazine
26 York Street
London W1U 6PZ
Tel: 020 7729 5454
Fax: 020 7739 0181
www.yogamagazine.co.uk

**Find Yoga+Joyful
Living magazine**
www.yimag.org

Yoga holidays
www.wellbeing
escapes.co.uk
www.yogaholidays.net

INDEX

Acknowledgements

The publishers would like to thank the following:

sweatyBetty for the loan of equipment featured. Visit their website for your nearest stockist www.sweatyBetty.com

Yogamatters for the loan of equipment featured.
For more information on their products, you can visit their website www.yogamatters.com

Sophy Ackroyd and Nicky Durrant for modelling the postures.